The Ultimate Fertility

Journal & Keepsake

An informative and easy-to-use
guide to help you get pregnant

By Alex & Elizabeth Lluch, Authors of Over 3 Million Books Sold!
and Dr. Benito Villanueva, OB-GYN and Reproductive Endocrinologist

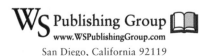

WS Publishing Group
www.WSPublishingGroup.com
San Diego, California 92119

The Ultimate Fertility Journal & Keepsake

By Alex & Elizabeth Lluch, Authors of Over 3 Million Books Sold!
and Dr. Benito Villanueva, OB-GYN and Reproductive Endocrinologist

Published by WS Publishing Group
San Diego, California 92119
Copyright © 2009 by WS Publishing Group

Design and Illustrations by:
David Defenbaugh, Sarah Jang
WS Publishing Group

For Inquiries:
Log on to www.WSPublishingGroup.com
E-mail info@WSPublishingGroup.com

ISBN 13: 978-1-934386-58-3

Printed in China

Table of Contents

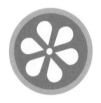

Introduction

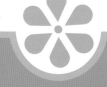

How to Use This Journal

The decision to have a baby and create a life is a monumental one for you and your partner. You may have uncovered this desire recently, or you may have been dreaming of being a parent your whole life. And, truly, becoming a mother or father is the greatest work you will ever do.

Naturally, conception is not the same journey for every couple. You probably have friends, family members, or coworkers who got pregnant after a few weeks or even days of trying. However, did you realize that it actually takes women an average of 8 months to conceive?

This book will help you understand the long list of factors that contribute to fertility and conception. Some are within your control, such as your weight or nutrition, and other factors — such as your age and family history — are not. This book will help you tackle the aspects of fertility that you can change and learn to best deal with those that are not in your control.

The Ultimate Fertility Journal & Keepsake will teach you the basics of ovulation and the top ways to boost your fertility for pregnancy success. This book provides you with 12 months of journal space, with 4 weeks in each month, to record the day of your monthly cycle, your basal body temperature, any vitamins you are taking, as well as your thoughts, hopes, and even worries. Each week is also full of interesting facts, tips for boosting fertility, fertility lingo explained, advice for looking ahead to pregnancy, and information just for dad to help keep you both educated, motivated, and in-tune with your body's every change.

Of course, millions of Americans find that getting pregnant is not such an easy road. If you try to conceive for more than a year — or if you try for 6 months and are over the age of 35 — you will want to get help from a medical professional.

In addition to a year's worth of journal pages, this book also offers a special section for couples working with fertility specialists, taking fertility medications, or employing IVF (in vitro fertilization). This book includes space to record the details of two full cycles of infertility treatments, including appointment dates, doses of oral and/or injectible medications, your doctor's special orders, and test results.

And because each cycle of IVF includes the dreaded Two-Week Wait after the embryo transfer, to determine if implantation was successful and you are pregnant, this book offers more journal space for venting your worries and hopes, replacing negative thoughts with positive ones, and writing about why you will make great parents. After all, if you do get pregnant, it will have all been worth the wait.

For some couples, the wait may be longer than for others. A year of trying may not be enough, and infertility treatments are not always successful for everyone. This book also includes a short section on what to do when you find yourselves asking, "What now?" From alternative medicine to adoption to taking a break and starting IVF again, your options for having a family are plentiful today.

> Every couple will have a different conception journey, but 8 months is the average amount of time it takes a woman to conceive.

Lastly, *The Ultimate Fertility Journal & Keepsake* closes by looking ahead to the first weeks after you discover you are, in fact, pregnant. For couples celebrating success, there will be much to do and know, so this section includes helpful tips for sharing the big news, as well as a checklist for early pregnancy.

Best of luck on your conception journey! Whatever path your journey takes you down, *The Ultimate Fertility Journal & Keepsake* will be your invaluable companion!

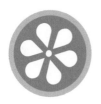

Fertility 101

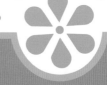

Fertility 101

Welcome to Fertility 101! Before you begin trying to conceive, there are a few things you need to do. Yes, just like any class, there is homework in Fertility 101.

There are several ways to boost your fertility and prepare for pregnancy, and the first is to let your physician know your plans. The preconception doctor's visit is vital, and you will want to come ready to discuss your personal and family medical history. This can help determine if there are any medical factors, such as diabetes or scarring from a sexually transmitted disease, that may inhibit the conception process. You will also go over the medications you are currently taking, and your doctor will let you know which are safe and which are off-limits during this important time.

> Your fertility involves a combination of factors — some that are within your control, such as your weight and diet, and others, such as your age and family history, which are not within your control.

And don't forget about the guys! Your partner should also have a checkup to make sure things are in working order and to circumvent any roadblocks to conception, such as being overweight (which may lower sperm count or concentration).

Of course, you will want to begin taking a prenatal vitamin or daily supplement of folic acid to prevent spina bifida and help your future baby's neural tube development. Don't wait until you get that positive pregnancy test to take a minimum of 400 micrograms of folic acid every day — important spinal cord development begins extremely early on in a pregnancy, and you will want to be prepared.

Your doctor's visit can also be a good time to discuss the effect your age will have on fertility. It's more common now for women to get pregnant well into their 40s, but it will be important to understand the role your age will play in conception. Each age group — 20s, 30s, and 40s — will have its own risks and ways to increase success.

And while you may not be able to change your past medical history or your age, there are lifestyle changes that can great improve your fertility and chances for conception. For instance, did you know that underweight and overweight women have a much tougher time getting pregnant? Being underweight or overweight can mean irregular periods or imbalanced estrogen levels, disrupting ovulation and making it difficult to conceive. If you fall into either category, talk to your doctor about an exercise and diet plan. Many times, gaining only a few pounds for underweight women, or losing just 5 to 10 percent of your body weight for overweight women, makes all the difference in conception.

> Every year in the United States, there are 60 million women considered to be of reproductive age.

Your eating habits will also affect fertility, so don't wait — start eating for pregnancy now. Skip the fad diets, which often mean you don't get the vitamins and minerals that you need, and beef up on whole grains, fruits and vegetables, and omega-3s (which come from olive oil, fortified eggs, and fish, such as salmon). On the flip side, you'll want to cut out bad fats, like trans fat, which is found in margarine and sugary food, which disrupts the way your body regulates insulin and can negatively affect fertility.

Next, if you're living a sedentary lifestyle — aka, you're a couch potato — it is time to get moving to jump-start your fertility. Just 30 minutes of moderate exercise a few times a week is enough to make a difference. If the gym isn't for you, purchase DVDs to work out at home. Or, get your partner involved and take a brisk walk together every night after dinner. The more you exercise now, the better off you will be during and after your pregnancy.

Clearly, a big part of Fertility 101 is lifestyle changes that are beneficial now, while you're trying to conceive, and later, when you are actually pregnant. For instance, morning and afternoon lattés may be part of your current daily routine, but a recent study by the *American Journal of Obstetrics and Gynecology* found that women who consumed 200 mg or more of caffeine daily (the equivalent of two cups of coffee or five cans of caffeinated soda) had twice the miscarriage risk of women who consumed no caffeine. Similarly, if you and dad enjoy a nightly alcoholic drink, you may find that now is the best time to cut back or quit entirely, since you will be going cold turkey once you are pregnant (and he may be joining you).

In 20 percent of women, ovulation does not trigger a rise in body temperature. Try combining an Ovulation Predictor Kit with monitoring your cervical mucus, in addition to charting your Basal Body Temperature.

And when it comes to smoking, it can't be stressed enough that you must quit now! The negative effects of smoking on fertility and pregnancy for both you and your partner are frightening. According to the American Society for Reproductive Medicine, they include an increase in impotence, miscarriage, and ectopic pregnancy, as well as low sperm count and an accelerated loss of eggs.

Eating right, exercising, and curbing bad habits will also help you reduce stress, which can contribute to trouble with fertility. Dr. Sarah Berga of Emory University School of Medicine has studied the impact of stress on fertility for years and concludes that while humans are designed to deal with a certain amount of stress, chronic stress may prevent some women from ovulating. Unfortunately, this can be a very stressful time for some couples! So, what can you do when people (who don't understand what you're going through) tell you, "Just relax and it will happen," instead of tearing your hair out? Try stress-reducers like yoga, meditation, deep breathing, walking, massage, or even acupuncture.

Finally, one of the most important parts of Fertility 101 is nurturing a healthy, happy relationship with your partner, throughout the ups and downs of the conception process. This means maintaining the spontaneity and intimacy in your sex life — even though the concept of "sex for procreation" isn't exactly sexy! This is also one of the best times to practice your communication skills, because you will both be experiencing a big range of emotions, from excitement and amazement to worry and fear, and will want to talk them out. Expressing why you want to be and will be good parents and offering unyielding support for one another helps you stay positive, excited, and motivated.

> There are about 6 million pregnancies in the U.S. each year.

Congratulations on your decision to become parents! As the lovable and wise Winnie the Pooh said, "A grand adventure is about to begin."

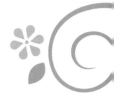

Stopping Birth Control

Stopping birth control can be as easy as not wearing a condom — or it may require a bit more calculation. It depends on the method you and your partner have been using, and for how long.

If your preferred method of birth control has been a barrier method, including condoms, you could get pregnant the very next time you have unprotected sex.

If you've been on the Pill, it is possible to ovulate in as early as two weeks after stopping, and your menstrual cycles should be regular again in as little as 3 months.

On the other hand, if you have been using an IUD (Intrauterine Device) it may take one full cycle after the device is removed before conception can be successful.

Understanding Ovulation

This journal is designed to help you chart your cycle for 12 months. When you're working to get pregnant, timing it so your egg and your partner's sperm meet and mingle is everything. Since sperm can live in the female body for 3 to 5 days, sex must occur during ovulation (when the ovary releases the egg) or a few days before ovulation. If the egg isn't fertilized, it breaks apart and leaves the body in the form of your menstrual period — and you'll have to wait to try again the next cycle. If you can't pinpoint the day of ovulation, you can take fertility specialists' suggestion and have sex every other day, although this can get exhausting. Luckily, there are a few techniques to help you determine when you are most fertile.

Track Your Cycle

Ovulation occurs two weeks before the start of your next period, so you can calculate it fairly accurately if you have a regular cycle and know the date of your upcoming period. However, the average woman's cycle lasts between 28 and 32 days, and it may be irregular from month to month due to stress or other factors. Recording your monthly cycle in the journal pages provided will help you get a feel for your most fertile days of each month.

Measure Your Basal Body Temperature

Basal body temperature (BBT) is your body's temperature as soon as you wake up in the morning — before doing anything, even going to the bathroom or brushing your teeth. An average woman's BBT is between 96 and 99 degrees Fahrenheit and will increase by about one-half of a degree when the ovary releases the egg.

Because this increase in body temperature is so tiny, you will need to buy a special basal thermometer (you can find one at the drugstore for about $10), and keep it at your bedside to ensure accurate readings, first thing in the morning. Do this at about the same time every day, beginning on the first day of your cycle, and record your BBT in the journal pages. You are most fertile and most likely to get pregnant two or three days before your temperature hits the highest point (which indicates ovulation) and 12 to 24 hours after ovulation.

Supplement an Ovulation Predictor Kit

You may find it useful to combine tracking your cycle and BBT with an Ovulation Predictor Kit (OPK) — an at-home test that pinpoints your fertile days by detecting the surge of luteinizing hormone (LH) that occurs just before ovulation. Once you see this surge, it's time! Have sex immediately!

It may seem like a lot to worry about at once, but tracking your BBT while using an OPK has dual benefits. Whereas a rise in your BBT often indicates that ovulation is almost over, an Ovulation Predictor Kit will indicate when ovulation is just beginning. By charting your BBT while using an OPK, you can see if your surge in luteinizing hormones corresponds with the rise in your basal temperature. Also, if you see that your BBT continues to remain high for two or three weeks after ovulation, this may mean you are pregnant!

There are several popular OPK brands that involve sticks or strips to test your urine, so check with your doctor to see which one he or she recommends.

Get Acquainted with Your Cervical Mucus

Forget being squeamish, because one of the best ways to accurately determine your window for peak fertility is by monitoring your cervical mucus. As your body nears ovulation, it starts producing a type of cervical mucus that is especially sperm-friendly (its job is to keep sperm alive for up to 5 days) and isn't seen at other times during your cycle. During your normal cycle, your cervical mucus will feel dry, but when you are at your peak fertility point, it will have a slippery, stickier consistency, often likened to egg whites.

You can monitor the look and feel of your cervical mucus when you find it in your underwear or by wiping with toilet paper. Also, if you like, insert a clean finger into the vagina, then gauge the consistency by stretching the cervical mucus out between your fingers. During your most fertile period, it may stretch up to several inches.

Just be sure not to confuse cervical mucus with semen. They can appear very similar, so always test before you have sex.

Five Myths About Fertility

Fertility doesn't have to do with the stars aligning or orgasm leading to spontaneous ovulation (where did that one come from?). There are many fertility myths floating around; here are a few of the most common ones, dispelled.

Myth 1: Ovulation occurs at Day 14.

Wouldn't that be convenient?! If it was that easy to figure out ovulation, getting pregnant would be a snap. In reality, the average woman's cycle is between 28 and 32 days, can be shorter or longer, and may differ from month to month. Your best bet is to have sex every other day or every day during the middle of your cycle to increase your chances of conception.

Myth 2: You should have sex every day to increase your chances of conceiving.

Actually, having sex every day can deplete your partner's sperm count, not to mention exhaust you both. Can you really expect to keep up the once-a-day for months? Fertility specialists recommend having sex every other day, and since sperm can live for up to 5 days inside your body, this is plenty.

Myth 3: You can spontaneously ovulate at any time.

Only one egg is released in each cycle, except in the rare instance that two are released within a 24-hour period of one another — if both are fertilized, it results in fraternal twins. Aside from multiple ovulation within that 24-hour window, a woman can't spontaneously ovulate at any time during her cycle, because the hormone progesterone suppresses the release of additional eggs after one is released in each cycle.

Myth 4: Stress causes infertility.

The true effect of stress on the ability to conceive has yet to be determined. Some studies show a definite link between chronic stress and difficulty conceiving; other studies show that the body is designed to tolerate outside stress, and so it should not affect fertility.

What is true is that stress certainly affects your mind, health, and the regularity of your menstrual cycle. You may notice that your period comes on an off-day during a month that you are particularly stressed out at work, for instance.

In actuality, infertility is a medical problem, and while managing stress can ease your conception journey, stress doesn't cause infertility.

Myth 5: Since you didn't have trouble conceiving with your first baby, this second pregnancy should be no problem.

Unfortunately, more than 1 million couples struggle with "secondary infertility," according to the National Survey of Family Growth. The fact of the matter is, you or your partner may have developed fertility issues since the last time you were pregnant. This can be anything from hormonal and sperm-production changes, to endometriosis, to weight gain and other lifestyle changes. Additionally, aging may play a part this time around. If it has been a few years since your last pregnancy, this can play a role in secondary infertility.

Luckily, secondary infertility is often less difficult to treat than primary infertility, since you and your doctor can pin down the changes in your body and lifestyle since the first pregnancy.

Trying Again After Miscarriage

It can be terrifying to learn that 15 to 25 percent of recognized pregnancies in the U.S. end in miscarriage; that's more than 1 million each year. And that number is really probably much higher, considering that many pregnancies end before the woman even knows she is pregnant (termed an "unrecognized pregnancy"). Fortunately, the chance of having two miscarriages in a row is less than 5 percent, and the likelihood of three is just 1 percent, according to the American Society for Reproductive Medicine.

Miscarriage does not indicate anything about your fertility. Chromosomal abnormalities in the fetus are responsible for 70 percent of miscarriages, and you may be comforted to know that the vast majority of women who have had a miscarriage go on to have healthy, full-term pregnancies.

If you've had a miscarriage, doctors usually suggest you wait 1 to 2 months, or until after you've had one normal menstrual cycle, before trying again. However, not all couples are emotionally ready that quickly. It is normal and expected that you grieve after suffering a miscarriage. Great hope and joy go into pregnancy, and when it ends unexpectedly, there is a profound sense of loss. You may not fully understand why or how this has happened, and others may have a hard time understanding your grief.

If you have had a miscarriage in the past, wait until you are ready, but understand that the chances of having a normal, healthy pregnancy are still very high for when you decide to try again.

Finally, there are many great counseling and support group options out there if you and your partner find that a previous miscarriage has caused depression or anxiety. Talk to your doctor about getting the support you need to help you along the road to conception.

Out-of-the-Box Fertility

More and more women are turning to complementary or alternative medicine and practices in hopes of boosting their fertility. While most evidence in support of these therapies is anecdotal and not scientifically proven, you may discover relaxation and stress-relieving benefits. For some women, these practices may make perfect sense, while others may think, "That's nuts!" Whatever camp you fall into, here are three less-conventional ideas that you might consider for revving up fertility.

Yoga

Yoga for fertility is a fast-growing trend that has spawned classes, DVDs, and postures designed specifically to stimulate the reproductive system and encourage fertility. Yoga is a 3,000-year-old practice that may benefit women trying to conceive by regulating hormone levels, reducing stress, increasing focus, and promoting relaxation using postures designed to restore and strengthen the body.

While the correlation between yoga and fertility isn't clearly defined, a 2002 Harvard Medical School study looked at 182 infertile women, a portion of whom participated in a relaxation and yoga program, while the others did not. The women in the yoga program were nearly three times more likely to get pregnant than the control group. *Namaste!*

Acupuncture

Acupuncture thrives on the idea that our bodies' energy, or chi, flows along pathways called meridians, and that inserting ultra-thin needles at specific points on these meridians can redirect or unblock the flow of energy. For example, acupuncturists claim to be able to redirect blood flow to the uterus or ovaries. In addition, weekly treatments of the 2,500-year-old Asian practice can reduce the stress that comes with trying to conceive.

Just be certain you find a trained acupuncturist, and that he or she not place needles in the abdominal or pelvic areas if you are being treated with IUI or IVF. You can find a licensed practitioner in your area by visiting the website for the National Certification Commission for Acupuncture and Oriental Medicine (www.nccaom.org).

Reiki

For the needle-shy, Reiki is a type of bodywork (think, super-lightweight massage therapy) in which the practitioner lays his or her hands on a client's body, while harnessing healthy chi outside of themselves and transferring it into the other person. According to The International Center for Reiki Training, "Reiki is a Japanese technique for stress reduction and relaxation that also promotes healing. If one's life force energy is low, then we are more likely to get sick or feel stress, and if it is high, we are more capable of being happy and healthy."

Reiki purports to clear blockages and create a state of inner peace and balance that paves the way for smooth conception. While the proof that Reiki aids fertility is purely anecdotal, many women enjoy its calming, restorative benefits. To find a Reiki pro, visit the International Association of Reiki Professionals at www.iarp.org.

My Fertility Diary

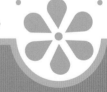

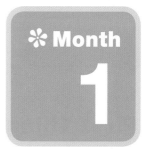

Month

1

"Go confidently in the direction of your dreams.
Live the life you have imagined."

~ Henry David Thoreau

Before
You Begin

Before you start your conception journey, your body needs to be primed for pregnancy. Even if you generally live a healthy lifestyle, there are several things you should do immediately to be best equipped to conceive, including taking folic acid, limiting exposure to hazardous chemicals, and thinking about switching to certain organic products. And since you may be pregnant in a matter of months, you will want to take one last opportunity to (safely) live it up. Think of this as prepping your body and lifestyle for your baby!

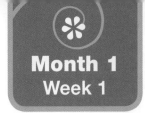

First Things First:
Folic Acid

Perhaps the most important first step you can take is loading up on folic acid, which is found in leafy greens, beans, fortified breads and cereal, and OJ. Start taking a multi- or prenatal vitamin with 400 micrograms of folic acid. The Centers for Disease Control reports that folic acid lowers your chances of having a baby with neural-tube defects like spina bifida by up to 70 percent.

✻ My Fertility Diary

• Monday

cycle day ⬜ basal body temp ⬜ vitamin ⬜

....
....
....

• Tuesday

cycle day ⬜ basal body temp ⬜ vitamin ⬜

....
....
....

• Wednesday

cycle day ⬜ basal body temp ⬜ vitamin ⬜

....
....
....

• Thursday

cycle day [____]   basal body temp [____]   vitamin [____]

....
....
....

• Friday

cycle day [____]   basal body temp [____]   vitamin [____]

....
....
....

• Saturday

cycle day [____]   basal body temp [____]   vitamin [____]

....
....
....

• Sunday

cycle day [____]   basal body temp [____]   vitamin [____]

....
....
....

My ✿ Thoughts

I first started thinking about having a baby ...

....
....
....
....
....
....
....
....
....
....
....
....

Daily ✿ Dangers

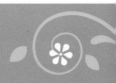

If your job exposes you to chemicals or radiation, you will need to work out a way to avoid these toxins. In addition, some potent cleaning supplies, insect repellents, paint products, and solvents may be harmful to your fertility and should be avoided.

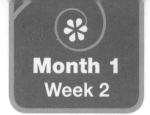

Month 1
Week 2

Food for Thought

There is some research that suggests that constant exposure to pesticides, herbicides, and additives in the food we eat can lead to reproductive problems. Pre-pregnancy is a great time to go organic, as commercially grown foods contain harmful chemicals that have been linked to cancer and other diseases. Organic products can be expensive, however, so if you have to prioritize, make the following items organic: milk, meat, nectarines, pears, peaches, apples, cherries, strawberries, grapes, spinach, potatoes, bell peppers, and raspberries.

❁ My Fertility Diary

• Monday

cycle day ⬭   basal body temp ⬭   vitamin ⬭

....
....
....

• Tuesday

cycle day ⬭   basal body temp ⬭   vitamin ⬭

....
....
....

• Wednesday

cycle day ⬭   basal body temp ⬭   vitamin ⬭

....
....
....

• Thursday

cycle day [ ] basal body temp [ ] vitamin [ ]

....
....
....

• Friday

cycle day [ ] basal body temp [ ] vitamin [ ]

....
....
....

• Saturday

cycle day [ ] basal body temp [ ] vitamin [ ]

....
....
....

• Sunday

cycle day [ ] basal body temp [ ] vitamin [ ]

....
....
....

My ❄ Thoughts

I think we will make good parents because …

....
....
....
....
....
....
....
....
....
....
....
....

Did You ❄ Know?

Sixty-year-old Frieda Birnbaum of New Jersey is the oldest woman to give birth to twins in the U.S. While there are no age limits on IVF treatments, the Society for Assisted Reproductive Technology recommends that women be under age 50 if they are undergoing IVF with a donor egg, and under 44 if they are using their own eggs.

27

Live It Up!

Now that you're thinking about getting pregnant, it's a good time to do, eat, and enjoy all the things that won't be available to you when you have a bun in the oven. If the daredevil in you has always wanted to skydive, now's the time. If you love sushi, eat up, since it will be off limits during pregnancy. Do you and your husband enjoy a good soak in the hot tub? Make this your last spa night for a while, since the high temperatures can decrease both of your fertility and can harm a fetus later on. And you may want to plan one final girls' night out (for the time being), since you'll want to cut out smoking and alcohol, starting now.

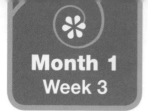

❋ My Fertility Diary

• Monday

cycle day ⬚   basal body temp ⬚   vitamin ⬚

• Tuesday

cycle day ⬚   basal body temp ⬚   vitamin ⬚

• Wednesday

cycle day ⬚   basal body temp ⬚   vitamin ⬚

• Thursday

cycle day [ ] basal body temp [ ] vitamin [ ]

....
....
....

• Friday

cycle day [ ] basal body temp [ ] vitamin [ ]

....
....
....

• Saturday

cycle day [ ] basal body temp [ ] vitamin [ ]

....
....
....

• Sunday

cycle day [ ] basal body temp [ ] vitamin [ ]

....
....
....

My ✿
Thoughts

Our biggest hope for our fertility journey is ...

....
....
....
....
....
....
....
....
....
....
....

Fertility ✿ Lingo

Can't keep all the acronyms straight? Here's a glossary of common shorthand you will see in this book and other resources you may read.

TTC: Trying to conceive
BBT: Basal body temperature
OPK: Ovulation Predictor Kit
CD: Cycle day
CM: Cervical mucus

HPT: Home pregnancy test
U/S: Ultrasound
PG: Pregnant
ART: Assisted Reproductive Technology or Technique

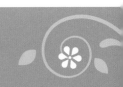

29

Just for Dad

Dad, you're one-half of this process, and not just when it comes to sex. In preparation for trying to conceive, you should get super-educated on fertility, diet and nutrition, and how you can help support mom during this time. You will want to understand everything she is doing to track ovulation, including taking her temperature, monitoring her body changes, and recording her cycle in this journal.

❋ My Fertility Diary

• Monday

cycle day ⬚   basal body temp ⬚   vitamin ⬚

....
....
....

• Tuesday

cycle day ⬚   basal body temp ⬚   vitamin ⬚

....
....
....

• Wednesday

cycle day ⬚   basal body temp ⬚   vitamin ⬚

....
....
....

• Thursday

cycle day [ ] basal body temp [ ] vitamin [ ]

....
....
....

• Friday

cycle day [ ] basal body temp [ ] vitamin [ ]

....
....
....

• Saturday

cycle day [ ] basal body temp [ ] vitamin [ ]

....
....
....

• Sunday

cycle day [ ] basal body temp [ ] vitamin [ ]

....
....
....

My Thoughts

Throughout our fertility journey, we will always ...

....
....
....
....
....
....
....
....
....
....
....
....

Questions to Consider

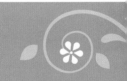

- What made us decide to start trying for a baby?
- Why do we feel we are prepared for a child?
- What are we most looking forward to about being parents?
- What is our number one question about conception?
- What is our biggest concern about pregnancy?

My Reflections

....
....
....
....
....
....
....
....
....
....
....
....
....
....
....
....
....
....
....
....
....
....
....

"Making the decision to have a child is momentous. It is to decide forever to have your heart go walking around outside your body."

~ Elizabeth Stone

Medical History Lesson

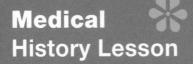

Once you're pregnant, it will seem like the doctor's office is your second home, but did you know that having preconception checkups are also crucial? Preconception appointments are designed to identify and reduce risk factors that might affect your pregnancy — including medical conditions, genetics, environmental toxins, and substance use — so that you can have the healthiest pregnancy and baby possible. You and your partner need to be very knowledgeable about your personal and family medical histories before this appointment, so make a list of questions and things to bring up before you go.

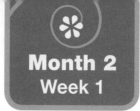

A Team Effort

First and foremost, your partner needs to attend your preconception doctor's appointment and genetic counseling sessions with you. You should be ready to talk about both of your medical histories, including preexisting conditions and illnesses, past pregnancies, social factors, and medications you take. Your doctor will need to know if you have had any past miscarriages or abortions. You should also discuss if either of you have any major risk factors, such as drug use or sexually transmitted diseases.

✽ My Fertility Diary

• Monday

cycle day ⬚   basal body temp ⬚   vitamin ⬚

• Tuesday

cycle day ⬚   basal body temp ⬚   vitamin ⬚

• Wednesday

cycle day ⬚   basal body temp ⬚   vitamin ⬚

• Thursday

cycle day [ ] basal body temp [ ] vitamin [ ]

....
....
....

• Friday

cycle day [ ] basal body temp [ ] vitamin [ ]

....
....
....

• Saturday

cycle day [ ] basal body temp [ ] vitamin [ ]

....
....
....

• Sunday

cycle day [ ] basal body temp [ ] vitamin [ ]

....
....
....

My ❀ Thoughts

One question we have for our doctor is ...

....
....
....
....
....
....
....
....
....
....
....
....
....
....

Look at Your ❀ Family Tree

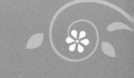

If any genetic or inheritable diseases run in your family, such as diabetes or muscular dystrophy, your doctor will refer you to a genetic counselor who can guide you on how to test for and minimize the risk of passing these diseases on to your future child.

Call Your Mother

You and your doctor will want to be aware of any potential roadblocks to conception now, and knowing your mother's reproductive and fertility history can help with this. Ask your mother, did she have an easy or difficult time conceiving? For instance, if she suffered from endometriosis, you are twice as likely to experience it as well. Your doctor will also be interested to know if she had any miscarriages or if there is a history of multiple births in your family.

❄ My Fertility Diary

• Monday

cycle day [   ]   basal body temp [   ]   vitamin [   ]

• Tuesday

cycle day [   ]   basal body temp [   ]   vitamin [   ]

• Wednesday

cycle day [   ]   basal body temp [   ]   vitamin [   ]

• Thursday

cycle day ☐   basal body temp ☐   vitamin ☐

....
....
....

• Friday

cycle day ☐   basal body temp ☐   vitamin ☐

....
....
....

• Saturday

cycle day ☐   basal body temp ☐   vitamin ☐

....
....
....

• Sunday

cycle day ☐   basal body temp ☐   vitamin ☐

....
....
....

My ❀ Thoughts

We are most nervous about ...

....
....
....
....
....
....
....
....
....
....
....
....
....
....

Questions ❀ for Your Doctor

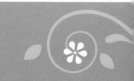

- Are my vaccinations up to date?
- Do I need to have my iron levels checked?
- Are there specific nutrient-rich foods I should start to include in my diet?
- Do I have any health problems that should be treated prior to trying to conceive?
- What kind of prenatal vitamin should I take?
- What are the initial signs of pregnancy I should look out for?

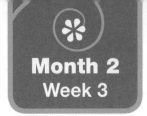

List Your
Medications

Some prescription, over-the-counter medications, herbs, vitamins, and supplements are not safe to take while you are trying to conceive or during pregnancy. Make a list of everything you take and bring it to your doctor during your preconception checkup.

....
....
....
....

❁ My Fertility Diary

• Monday

cycle day ⬭   basal body temp ⬭   vitamin ⬭
....
....
....

• Tuesday

cycle day ⬭   basal body temp ⬭   vitamin ⬭
....
....
....

• Wednesday

cycle day ⬭   basal body temp ⬭   vitamin ⬭
....
....
....

• Thursday

cycle day ◻ basal body temp ◻ vitamin ◻

....
....
....

• Friday

cycle day ◻ basal body temp ◻ vitamin ◻

....
....
....

• Saturday

cycle day ◻ basal body temp ◻ vitamin ◻

....
....
....

• Sunday

cycle day ◻ basal body temp ◻ vitamin ◻

....
....
....

My ❄
Thoughts

We are
most excited
about ...

....
....
....
....
....
....
....
....
....
....
....
....
....
....

Did ❄
You Know?

Did you realize that periodontal disease has been linked to miscarriage and other pregnancy complications, such as premature labor? You should make an appointment with your dentist to have your teeth and gums checked now.

Month 2
Week 4

Being Frank

If you or your partner has ever had a sexually transmitted disease, you *must* speak up when you meet with your doctor. STDs like Chlamydia and gonorrhea, when left untreated, can lead to infertility and ectopic pregnancy. While it may be embarrassing or scary to discuss this, being honest and frank can save your pregnancy. According to the Centers for Disease Control, STDs are one of the most preventable causes of infertility.

My Fertility Diary

• Monday

cycle day | basal body temp | vitamin

• Tuesday

cycle day | basal body temp | vitamin

• Wednesday

cycle day | basal body temp | vitamin

• Thursday

cycle day | basal body temp | vitamin

....

....

....

• Friday

cycle day | basal body temp | vitamin

....

....

....

....

• Saturday

cycle day | basal body temp | vitamin

....

....

....

....

• Sunday

cycle day | basal body temp | vitamin

....

....

....

....

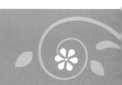

My Thoughts

What does being parents mean to us?

....

....

....

....

....

....

....

....

....

....

....

....

....

....

Fertility Lingo

Hx: history, particularly medical
Dx: diagnosis
Tx: treatment
Rx: prescription

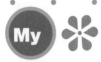

My Reflections

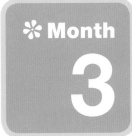

Month 3

"The question isn't who is going to let me,
it's who is going to stop me."

~ Ayn Rand

Age: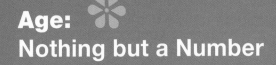
Nothing but a Number

With modern fertility treatments, such as egg donation and in vitro fertilization, and a deeper understanding of conception, there has never been a better time to get pregnant, no matter your age. In fact, in recent years, more babies were born to women between ages 30 and 35 than to any other age group! Women well into their 40s — and even 50s — are conceiving and giving birth to healthy, happy babies. There are, of course, helpful ways to maximize success and minimize risks at every age, so read on!

Month 3
Week 1

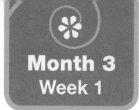

Fertility in Your Twenties

Your 20s are obviously the most fertile time in your life, with the lowest risk for complications. According to the American Society for Reproductive Medicine, less than 10 percent of women in their 20s struggle with infertility. In your early 20s, the chances of conceiving within one year of trying are about 98 percent, dipping to 84 percent by your late-20s. In addition, the pregnancy success rate is 20 to 25 percent for each ovulation cycle.

My Fertility Diary

• Monday

cycle day ______ basal body temp ______ vitamin ______

• Tuesday

cycle day ______ basal body temp ______ vitamin ______

• Wednesday

cycle day ______ basal body temp ______ vitamin ______

• Thursday

cycle day [ ]   basal body temp [ ]   vitamin [ ]

....
....
....

• Friday

cycle day [ ]   basal body temp [ ]   vitamin [ ]

....
....
....

• Saturday

cycle day [ ]   basal body temp [ ]   vitamin [ ]

....
....
....

• Sunday

cycle day [ ]   basal body temp [ ]   vitamin [ ]

....
....
....

My Thoughts

If we could choose, we would have ____ children, ____ boy(s) and ____ girl(s). Why?

....
....
....
....
....
....
....
....
....
....
....

Did You Know?

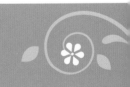

All females are born with 1 million eggs — all the eggs they will have in their lifetime, although only about 300 will be released during the reproductive years. As women age, the number of healthy eggs the ovaries produce declines, dropping off sharply around age 35. And after age 45, studies show that the ability to get pregnant using your own eggs drops to about 1 percent — in that case, donor eggs are a viable option with good rates of success.

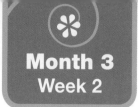

The Thirties:
Pregnancy Primetime

Although your fertility begins to dip in your mid-30s, many people consider this age the perfect time to get pregnant, because you are likely to be more stable in your relationship, career, and financial situation than in your 20s. In your 30s, you have a 15 percent chance of getting pregnant during any cycle, and your chances of conceiving within a year are 65 to 75 percent.

❋ My Fertility Diary

• Monday

cycle day   basal body temp   vitamin

• Tuesday

cycle day   basal body temp   vitamin

• Wednesday

cycle day   basal body temp   vitamin

• Thursday

cycle day [ ] basal body temp [ ] vitamin [ ]

....
....
....

• Friday

cycle day [ ] basal body temp [ ] vitamin [ ]

....
....
....

• Saturday

cycle day [ ] basal body temp [ ] vitamin [ ]

....
....
....

• Sunday

cycle day [ ] basal body temp [ ] vitamin [ ]

....
....
....

My ❀ Thoughts

My biggest concern about my fertility is ...

....
....
....
....
....
....
....
....
....
....
....
....
....

Twins ❀ in Your Thirties

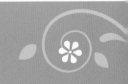

Women age 35 to 39 are more likely to have twins than any other age group, even without using fertility treatments that increase the likelihood of having multiples. This is because, as you age, FSH (follicle stimulating hormone) levels increase, upping the chance of the ovaries releasing multiple eggs during one cycle.

Fabulous Forties

Once a woman passes age 40, her chances for conceiving during an ovulation cycle drop significantly, to just 5 percent. Infertility in older women may be due to a higher risk of chromosomal abnormalities in the eggs as they age. However, by using fertility treatments like IVF, the chance of success using donor eggs is high — greater than 50 percent. Interestingly, women in their 40s are more apt to breast-feed and make healthier nutritional choices during pregnancy, according to a study published in the *Journal of the American Dietetic Association*.

✻ My Fertility Diary

• Monday

cycle day ⬚   basal body temp ⬚   vitamin ⬚

• Tuesday

cycle day ⬚   basal body temp ⬚   vitamin ⬚

• Wednesday

cycle day ⬚   basal body temp ⬚   vitamin ⬚

• Thursday

cycle day [ ]   basal body temp [ ]   vitamin [ ]

....
....
....

• Friday

cycle day [ ]   basal body temp [ ]   vitamin [ ]

....
....
....

• Saturday

cycle day [ ]   basal body temp [ ]   vitamin [ ]

....
....
....

• Sunday

cycle day [ ]   basal body temp [ ]   vitamin [ ]

....
....
....

My ❋ Thoughts

Characteristics we hope our baby inherits from me include ...

....
....
....
....
....
....
....
....
....
....
....
....

Fertility ❋ Lingo

FSH: follicle stimulating hormone, which stimulates the ovaries to produce an egg for fertilization

Follicular atresia: the natural process throughout the course of a woman's reproductive life in which thousands of her immature eggs, or follicles, will fail to become eggs and die

Just for Dad

Although men don't experience the same drastic fertility drop-off as women, male fertility also decreases with each passing decade, including lessened sperm count and reduced motility of the sperm (meaning they're worse swimmers than before). The best ways to prevent fertility loss in men are with regular exercise and a healthy diet of fresh foods.

❋ My Fertility Diary

• Monday

cycle day [ ]   basal body temp [ ]   vitamin [ ]

....
....
....

• Tuesday

cycle day [ ]   basal body temp [ ]   vitamin [ ]

....
....
....

• Wednesday

cycle day [ ]   basal body temp [ ]   vitamin [ ]

....
....
....

• Thursday

cycle day [   ] basal body temp [   ] vitamin [   ]

....
....
....

• Friday

cycle day [   ] basal body temp [   ] vitamin [   ]

....
....
....

• Saturday

cycle day [   ] basal body temp [   ] vitamin [   ]

....
....
....

• Sunday

cycle day [   ] basal body temp [   ] vitamin [   ]

....
....
....

My

Thoughts

Characteristics we hope our baby inherits from dad include ...

....

....

....

....

....

....

....

....

....

....

....

....

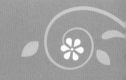

Questions ✾ for Your Doctor

- What kinds of fertility risks are associated with my age group?
- What can I do to minimize risks?
- What can I do if my periods are not regular?
- How long should we try before we consult an infertility specialist?

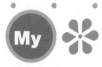

My Reflections

....
....
....
....
....
....
....
....
....
....
....
....
....
....
....
....
....
....
....
....
....
....
....
....
....

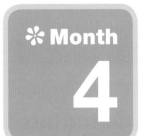

"Be content upon the perfection
of the present day."

~ William Law

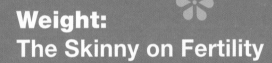

Weight:
The Skinny on Fertility

You've heard all about how much weight
you're meant to gain during pregnancy,
but, actually, your weight plays a big role in
helping you conceive, as well. Studies have
shown that women who are underweight or
overweight have a significantly more difficult
time getting pregnant. Luckily, gaining a
few pounds or losing just 5 to 10 percent of
your body weight can dramatically improve
your chances of getting pregnant — not
to mention reducing your risk of diabetes,
high blood pressure, and heart disease, and
boosting your self-esteem!

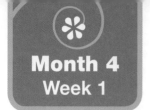

Calculate Your BMI

Get a calculator and use this formula to find your BMI:

(Lbs. / [Height in inches^2]) x 703

Your BMI:

....

What does your BMI mean?

- Less than 18.5: underweight
- 18.5 – 24.9: ideal weight
- 25 to 29.9: overweight
- 30 and above: obese

✳ My Fertility Diary

• Monday

cycle day ⬜   basal body temp ⬜   vitamin ⬜

....
....
....

• Tuesday

cycle day ⬜   basal body temp ⬜   vitamin ⬜

....
....
....

• Wednesday

cycle day ⬜   basal body temp ⬜   vitamin ⬜

....
....
....

• Thursday

cycle day [   ]   basal body temp [   ]   vitamin [   ]

....
....
....

• Friday

cycle day [   ]   basal body temp [   ]   vitamin [   ]

....
....
....

• Saturday

cycle day [   ]   basal body temp [   ]   vitamin [   ]

....
....
....

• Sunday

cycle day [   ]   basal body temp [   ]   vitamin [   ]

....
....
....

My Thoughts

When I think about my weight, I feel ...

....
....
....
....
....
....
....
....
....
....
....
....
....
....

Did You Know?

Twelve percent of all infertility cases are a result of a woman either weighing too little or too much. The American Society for Reproductive Medicine reports this is because overweight women produce too much estrogen (a sex hormone produced in fat cells), which acts as natural birth control. On the flip side, a woman with too little body fat can't produce enough estrogen and her cycle may become irregular or even shut down.

55

Your
Weight Profile

Your BMI indicates that you are ...
❑ an ideal weight ❑ overweight ❑ underweight

What is your percentage of body fat? ....

How steady is your weight? Does it fluctuate often? Do you diet?
....

What types of diets have you tried? Any fad diets?
....

Do you plan to lose or gain weight to increase your chances of conception?
....

❋ My Fertility Diary

• Monday

cycle day ⬚   basal body temp ⬚   vitamin ⬚
....
....
....

• Tuesday

cycle day ⬚   basal body temp ⬚   vitamin ⬚
....
....
....

• Wednesday

cycle day ⬚   basal body temp ⬚   vitamin ⬚
....
....
....

• Thursday

cycle day [   ]   basal body temp [   ]   vitamin [   ]

....
....
....

• Friday

cycle day [   ]   basal body temp [   ]   vitamin [   ]

....
....
....
....

• Saturday

cycle day [   ]   basal body temp [   ]   vitamin [   ]

....
....
....

• Sunday

cycle day [   ]   basal body temp [   ]   vitamin [   ]

....
....
....

My ❁ Thoughts

The healthiest weight for me would be ...

....
....
....
....
....
....
....
....
....
....
....
....
....
....

Fertility ❁ Lingo

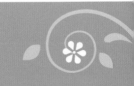

PCOS: Polycystic Ovarian Syndrome, a hormonal disorder affecting 6 to 8 percent of women of reproductive age, and a leading cause of infertility. Overweight women may be more likely to develop PCOS.

Just for Dad

Women aren't the only ones whose fertility is negatively affected by being overweight. Overweight men have lower sperm count, concentration, and quality. One U.S. study found that overweight men had a five-fold reduction in their sperm count compared to those of an average weight. If either of you are overweight, talk to your doctor about how you can both lose a few pounds in a healthy way.

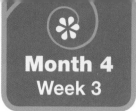

❋ My Fertility Diary

• Monday

cycle day ☐ basal body temp ☐ vitamin ☐

• Tuesday

cycle day ☐ basal body temp ☐ vitamin ☐

• Wednesday

cycle day ☐ basal body temp ☐ vitamin ☐

• Thursday

cycle day [ ]   basal body temp [ ]   vitamin [ ]

....
....
....

• Friday

cycle day [ ]   basal body temp [ ]   vitamin [ ]

....
....
....

• Saturday

cycle day [ ]   basal body temp [ ]   vitamin [ ]

....
....
....

• Sunday

cycle day [ ]   basal body temp [ ]   vitamin [ ]

....
....
....

My ❀ Thoughts

One thing we could do to be healthier is ...

....
....
....
....
....
....
....
....
....
....
....
....

Food ❀ for Thought

No matter how much weight you wind up gaining during pregnancy, you should never consider dieting. You will actually want to up your caloric intake by about 300 calories a day when you have a bun in the oven. Dieting is unsafe for your baby in that fat-burning diets produce a byproduct called ketones, which, in high quantities, have been linked to mental retardation. So skip the low-carb diet until after the baby is born.

Your Pregnant Future:
Pregnancy Weight Gain

Your pregnancy weight gain should be fairly slow and steady. Doctors say that, as a rule, women should gain 2 to 4 pounds during the first trimester, and then an additional 3 to 4 pounds per month during the second and third trimesters. The American College of Obstetricians and Gynecologists recommends a weight gain of 25 to 37 pounds for women who were a normal weight before pregnancy. Here is a breakdown of approximately how a 30-pound gain is distributed:

- 7½ pounds is the baby
- 1½ pounds is the placenta
- 4 pounds is attributed to increased fluid volume
- 2 pounds is the weight of the uterus
- 2 pounds is the weight of breast tissue
- 4 pounds is because of increased blood volume
- 7 pounds is attributed to stores of fat, protein and nutrients
- 2 pounds is the amniotic fluid

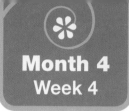

✴ My Fertility Diary

• Monday

cycle day ☐   basal body temp ☐   vitamin ☐

....
....
....

• Tuesday

cycle day ☐   basal body temp ☐   vitamin ☐

....
....
....

• Wednesday

cycle day ☐   basal body temp ☐   vitamin ☐

....
....
....

• Thursday

cycle day ⬚   basal body temp ⬚   vitamin ⬚

....
....
....

• Friday

cycle day ⬚   basal body temp ⬚   vitamin ⬚

....
....
....

• Saturday

cycle day ⬚   basal body temp ⬚   vitamin ⬚

....
....
....

• Sunday

cycle day ⬚   basal body temp ⬚   vitamin ⬚

....
....
....

My ✿ Thoughts

Am I apprehensive about gaining weight during pregnancy?

....
....
....
....
....
....
....
....
....
....
....
....

Questions ✿ for Your Doctor

- Is my body-fat ratio optimized for conception?
- Should I gain or lose weight to help my chances of getting pregnant?
- If so, how much weight?
- What are some easy and safe ways I can gain or lose a bit of weight?

My Reflections

....
....
....
....
....
....
....
....
....
....
....
....
....
....
....
....
....
....
....
....
....
....
....
....

"Life is magic, the way nature works
seems to be quite magical."
~ Jonas Salk

Your Pre-Pregnancy Diet

Not only does developing well-rounded eating habits help you conceive, but they will keep you and your baby healthy and happy when you do get pregnant. Plus, it will be easier to adjust to a healthy diet if you start eating for pregnancy now, instead of when you're in the thick of it. Just imagine trying to silence your sweet tooth when you're in the midst of pregnancy cravings, or forcing down broccoli when you're completely nauseous. It's never too early to practice eating for two! In addition, check with your doctor to see what vitamins and supplements can boost your fertility and prep you for pregnancy.

Nix
Trans Fats

Trans fats are found in commercial baked goods, fried food, margarine, and some prepackaged snack foods, and should be avoided when trying to conceive. A study from the Harvard School of Public Health followed 18,555 healthy women who were trying to get pregnant over an eight-year period; the results showed that participants who ate the most trans fats were the most likely to develop ovulatory infertility. The best way to completely cut out trans fats is to avoid hydrogenated or partially hydrogenated oils.

❖ My Fertility Diary

• Monday

cycle day ▢   basal body temp ▢   vitamin ▢

• Tuesday

cycle day ▢   basal body temp ▢   vitamin ▢

• Wednesday

cycle day ▢   basal body temp ▢   vitamin ▢

• Thursday

cycle day [ ]   basal body temp [ ]   vitamin [ ]

....
....
....

• Friday

cycle day [ ]   basal body temp [ ]   vitamin [ ]

....
....
....

• Saturday

cycle day [ ]   basal body temp [ ]   vitamin [ ]

....
....
....

• Sunday

cycle day [ ]   basal body temp [ ]   vitamin [ ]

....
....
....

My ❋ Thoughts

My favorite "bad" food is ...

....
....
....
....
....
....
....
....
....
....
....
....
....

Did You ❋ Know?

Getting 15 milligrams of zinc a day can help keep your reproductive system primed. The American Pregnancy Association reports that zinc contributes to ovulation and fertility in women and to semen and testosterone production in men; thus, deficiencies in zinc may hinder both female and male fertility. Try eating foods like oysters, which contain very high levels of zinc.

Your Pregnant Future:
Eating a Balanced Diet

According to the American College of Obstetricians and Gynecologists, pregnant women should have 3 servings of milk, yogurt, and cheese; 3 servings of protein; 3 servings of fruits; 4 servings of vegetables; and 9 servings of whole grain products each day. Make a list of your favorite foods in each category here.

Dairy:

Protein:

Fruits:

Vegetables:

Whole grains:

❈ My Fertility Diary

• Monday

cycle day ☐   basal body temp ☐   vitamin ☐

• Tuesday

cycle day ☐   basal body temp ☐   vitamin ☐

• Wednesday

cycle day ☐   basal body temp ☐   vitamin ☐

• Thursday

cycle day [ ]   basal body temp [ ]   vitamin [ ]

....
....
....

• Friday

cycle day [ ]   basal body temp [ ]   vitamin [ ]

....
....
....

• Saturday

cycle day [ ]   basal body temp [ ]   vitamin [ ]

....
....
....

• Sunday

cycle day [ ]   basal body temp [ ]   vitamin [ ]

....
....
....

My ❋ Thoughts

One fertility-boosting food I will add to my diet is ...

....
....
....
....
....
....
....
....
....
....
....
....
....

Fertility ❋ Lingo

Ovarian follicle: fluid-filled sacs where eggs develop and are released during ovulation

Ovarian reserve: a woman's supply of healthy eggs and thus, an indication of her fertility

Food for Thought

Women trying to conceive should get at least 1,000 mg of calcium a day — the amount in about 3 glasses of skim milk. Once pregnant, calcium is crucial to your growing baby's teeth and bones (and if you don't take in enough, your body will start drawing it from your own bones!). Get calcium from cottage cheese, low-fat yogurt and cheese, canned salmon, and rice, or start taking a supplement.

❋ My Fertility Diary

• Monday

cycle day ⬚ basal body temp ⬚ vitamin ⬚

....
....
....

• Tuesday

cycle day ⬚ basal body temp ⬚ vitamin ⬚

....
....
....

• Wednesday

cycle day ⬚ basal body temp ⬚ vitamin ⬚

....
....
....

• Thursday

cycle day [ ] basal body temp [ ] vitamin [ ]

....
....
....

• Friday

cycle day [ ] basal body temp [ ] vitamin [ ]

....
....
....

• Saturday

cycle day [ ] basal body temp [ ] vitamin [ ]

....
....
....

• Sunday

cycle day [ ] basal body temp [ ] vitamin [ ]

....
....
....

My ❀ Thoughts

One healthy treat I can reward myself with is ...

....
....
....
....
....
....
....
....
....
....
....
....
....

Iron ❀ Woman

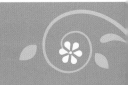

Anemia, or low red blood cell count, is a scary problem many pregnant women encounter. Prevent anemia now by beefing up on iron-rich foods, such as red meat, beans, pumpkin seeds, potatoes with skin, and fortified cereals. Also, remember how important it is take your prenatal vitamins daily.

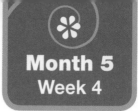

Just for Dad

Did you know dad's fertility can benefit from a multivitamin, male fertility supplement, or even a pre-natal vitamin? The antioxidants, vitamins, and minerals are said to improve sperm quality, count, and motility. Check with your doctor to see what he or she recommends.

❊ My Fertility Diary

• Monday

cycle day ( )   basal body temp ( )   vitamin ( )

• Tuesday

cycle day ( )   basal body temp ( )   vitamin ( )

• Wednesday

cycle day ( )   basal body temp ( )   vitamin ( )

• Thursday

cycle day [   ] basal body temp [   ] vitamin [   ]

....
....
....

• Friday

cycle day [   ] basal body temp [   ] vitamin [   ]

....
....
....

• Saturday

cycle day [   ] basal body temp [   ] vitamin [   ]

....
....
....

• Sunday

cycle day [   ] basal body temp [   ] vitamin [   ]

....
....
....

My Thoughts

The hardest food for me to give up during pregnancy will be ...

....
....
....
....
....
....
....
....
....
....
....

Questions for Your Doctor

- How much water do I need to drink every day to stay hydrated?
- I don't like to eat _____ (red meat, fish, green vegetables, etc.). Is there a supplement I can take to get the proper nutrients?
- I made of list of my favorite foods and drinks. Are there any I should cut back on or cut out of my diet completely?
- What are healthy treats I can have to reward myself or when I crave sweets?

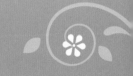

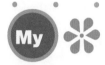

My Reflections

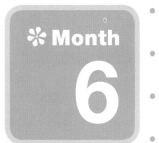

"We can do no great things;
only small things with great love."
~ Mother Teresa

Get Physical

Experts agree that 30 minutes of moderate exercise three or four times a week heightens fertility, as well as promotes a smooth pregnancy, easier delivery, and faster return to your pre-pregnancy size after the baby is born. Better still, no gym membership is necessary! You might try walking, swimming, bicycling, aerobics, or yoga, all of which relieve stress, burn fat (an enemy of conception), and get your heart rate up to a safe level. Just stick to a moderate workout routine (this isn't the time to train for a marathon, for instance); over-exercise is a major cause of infertility in women. And, of course, always check with your doctor before starting any exercise program.

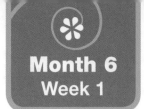

Get Motivated, Get Moving!

How many days each week do you do something physical? For how long each day? ....

Stop making excuses! Write down your top excuses for skipping exercise, then write down solutions. For instance, if you say, "I don't have time to exercise," the solution might be, "Use half of my lunch break to take a walk."

excuses: solutions:

....

....

....

....

❋ My Fertility Diary

• Monday

cycle day ⬚   basal body temp ⬚   vitamin ⬚

....

....

....

• Tuesday

cycle day ⬚   basal body temp ⬚   vitamin ⬚

....

....

....

• Wednesday

cycle day ⬚   basal body temp ⬚   vitamin ⬚

....

....

....

• Thursday

cycle day [ ]   basal body temp [ ]   vitamin [ ]

....
....
....

• Friday

cycle day [ ]   basal body temp [ ]   vitamin [ ]

....
....
....

• Saturday

cycle day [ ]   basal body temp [ ]   vitamin [ ]

....
....
....

• Sunday

cycle day [ ]   basal body temp [ ]   vitamin [ ]

....
....
....

My Thoughts

Types of exercise I enjoy include ...

....
....
....
....
....
....
....
....
....
....
....
....
....
....

Maintain a ❁ Workout Plan

Low-impact activities like swimming, walking, elliptical and stair-climbing machines, jogging, and yoga are things you can start doing now and safely continue throughout pregnancy. Exercise will also help ease some pregnancy symptoms and discomforts, such as back pain, swelling, and fatigue.

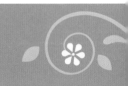

Keep
It Cool

Raising your core body temperature above 102 degrees Fahrenheit has been linked to birth defects and miscarriage, so you will want to avoid activities like Bikram (hot) yoga while you are trying to conceive. Ask your doctor if the intensity level of your workouts is keeping your heart rate and body temperature at a safe level — some experts believe that women trying to conceive should keep their heart rates under 140 beats per minute.

❁ My Fertility Diary

• Monday

cycle day ☐   basal body temp ☐   vitamin ☐

• Tuesday

cycle day ☐   basal body temp ☐   vitamin ☐

• Wednesday

cycle day ☐   basal body temp ☐   vitamin ☐

• Thursday

cycle day	basal body temp	vitamin

....
....
....

• Friday

cycle day	basal body temp	vitamin

....
....
....

• Saturday

cycle day	basal body temp	vitamin

....
....
....

• Sunday

cycle day	basal body temp	vitamin

....
....
....

My ✿
Thoughts

Types of exercise I can't stand include ...

....
....
....
....
....
....
....
....
....
....
....
....
....
....

Your ✿
Pregnant Future

There are certain sports and types of exercise you will have to avoid while pregnant. Activities that could cause you to fall or might result in abdominal trauma — horseback riding, ice skating, gymnastics, and skiing, for instance — are out of the question. You will also have to avoid scuba diving, as your developing baby won't be able to decompress safely.

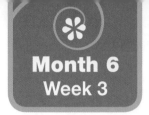

Just for Dad

While exercise is important for dad's fertility, he should be careful to keep his testicles from getting overheated. Sperm need to be kept cooler than his body temperature — around 92 or 93 degrees. He should avoid prolonged bicycle riding or other excessive exercise and try to stay away from tight underwear. Wearing boxers instead of briefs or boxer briefs will keep sperm cool and happy.

❊ My Fertility Diary

• Monday

cycle day ⬭   basal body temp ⬭   vitamin ⬭

....
....
....

• Tuesday

cycle day ⬭   basal body temp ⬭   vitamin ⬭

....
....
....

• Wednesday

cycle day ⬭   basal body temp ⬭   vitamin ⬭

....
....
....

• Thursday

cycle day [ ]   basal body temp [ ]   vitamin [ ]

....

....

....

• Friday

cycle day [ ]   basal body temp [ ]   vitamin [ ]

....

....

....

• Saturday

cycle day [ ]   basal body temp [ ]   vitamin [ ]

....

....

....

• Sunday

cycle day [ ]   basal body temp [ ]   vitamin [ ]

....

....

....

My ✽ Thoughts

The top things that motivate me to exercise are ...

....

....

....

....

....

....

....

....

....

....

....

....

Fertility ✽ Lingo

hCG: human Chorionic Gonadotropin, the hormone emitted by the human placenta, is what is measured during a pregnancy test. Medications that are comprised of hCG may be given during Assisted Reproductive Therapy.

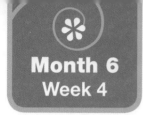

Amazing Abdominals

The two muscle groups that are most important during pregnancy are the abdominals and the pelvic floor. Having strong abs supports your back, which is under plenty of stress during pregnancy. Additionally, strengthening your abs can ease labor and delivery. So mix in a few crunches with each workout session. Or, consider yoga and Pilates, which both work the core muscles.

❋ My Fertility Diary

• Monday

cycle day [ ] basal body temp [ ] vitamin [ ]

• Tuesday

cycle day [ ] basal body temp [ ] vitamin [ ]

• Wednesday

cycle day [ ] basal body temp [ ] vitamin [ ]

• Thursday

cycle day [ ]   basal body temp [ ]   vitamin [ ]

....
....
....

• Friday

cycle day [ ]   basal body temp [ ]   vitamin [ ]

....
....
....

• Saturday

cycle day [ ]   basal body temp [ ]   vitamin [ ]

....
....
....

• Sunday

cycle day [ ]   basal body temp [ ]   vitamin [ ]

....
....
....

My Thoughts

Having a great workout makes me feel ...

....
....
....
....
....
....
....
....
....
....
....
....
....

Did You Know?

One of the best ways to stick to an exercise plan is to find a workout buddy — someone who has the same habits and goals as you. Also, pairing up someone whom you see every day, such as your partner, a coworker, or a neighbor, will make you more likely to stay motivated on days when you're feeling lazy.

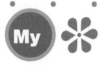

My Reflections

....
....
....
....
....
....
....
....
....
....
....
....
....
....
....
....
....
....
....
....
....
....

> "Where there is love, there is life."
> ~ Gandhi

Let's Talk About ... Sex ❋

When you're having sex for procreation, it can definitely feel like intimacy and passion go out the window. Thus, one of the most crucial parts of the conception journey is nurturing your relationship with dad and practicing your much-needed communication skills. Just because you're trying to conceive, doesn't mean you can't still plan date nights, be romantic, and make sex fun. After all, this process isn't only about getting pregnant; it's also about building the groundwork for your growing family.

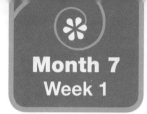

Month 7
Week 1

Talk
It Out

Communicating with dad can help you find some perspective and humor in this process. Be honest and open about how you're both feeling, emotionally and physically. You may be surprised to find out that you're experiencing the same nervousness or frustration. This is definitely a stressful time for many couples, but you have to be able to laugh at things like marking your "sex schedule" on a calendar.

✿ My Fertility Diary

• Monday

cycle day   basal body temp   vitamin

• Tuesday

cycle day   basal body temp   vitamin

• Wednesday

cycle day   basal body temp   vitamin

• Thursday

cycle day ⬚   basal body temp ⬚   vitamin ⬚

....
....
....

• Friday

cycle day ⬚   basal body temp ⬚   vitamin ⬚

....
....
....

• Saturday

cycle day ⬚   basal body temp ⬚   vitamin ⬚

....
....
....

• Sunday

cycle day ⬚   basal body temp ⬚   vitamin ⬚

....
....
....

My ❀ Thoughts

Scheduling sex to conceive makes us feel ...

....
....
....
....
....
....
....
....
....
....
....
....
....

Sex ❀ Should Be Sexy

Do your best to keep sex from feeling like a chore. Although it's impossible not to schedule sex during this time, you can still make it feel sexy and fun. Instead of saying, "I'm ovulating; we have to have sex tonight," try saying something like, "I've been thinking about how sexy you are all day, and I can't wait until you get home."

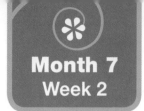

Make a Date

There are lots of ways to make time as a couple (some examples are below). Make a list of a few fun date ideas.

Romantic (enjoy a candlelight dinner or see a play):

....

Outdoorsy (pack a picnic or take a hike):

....

Playful (play board games or Frisbee):

....

Cultural (take a cooking class or visit a museum):

....

❈ My Fertility Diary

• **Monday**

cycle day ☐   basal body temp ☐   vitamin ☐

....
....
....

• **Tuesday**

cycle day ☐   basal body temp ☐   vitamin ☐

....
....
....

• **Wednesday**

cycle day ☐   basal body temp ☐   vitamin ☐

....
....
....

• Thursday

cycle day		basal body temp		vitamin	

....
....
....

• Friday

cycle day		basal body temp		vitamin	

....
....
....
....

• Saturday

cycle day		basal body temp		vitamin	

....
....
....

• Sunday

cycle day		basal body temp		vitamin	

....
....
....
....

My ❄ Thoughts

The last time we had a date, we ...

....
....
....
....
....
....
....
....
....
....
....
....
....
....
....

Plan ❄ a Getaway

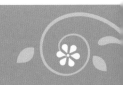

Many times, a quick, intimate getaway is all you need to recharge your sexual appetite or break out of a rut. Plan a weekend at a bed-and-breakfast. Ignore work responsibilities and shut out all distractions, including email, cell phones, and TV. Relax and enjoy each other's company — schedule a couple's massage, order room service, and sleep in. A change of scenery will inspire passion and relieve some of the stress of results-driven sex. You'll head back to reality feeling refreshed, energized, and sexually rejuvenated.

87

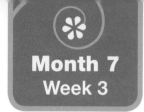

Month 7
Week 3

Your Pregnant Future

Unless your doctor warns you against it because of risk of complications, sex and orgasm will be safe during pregnancy. Certain positions may be more comfortable than others, but the baby will be fully protected by the fluid-filled amniotic sac. Additionally, a dense mucus plug seals off your cervix to keep out any infections.

❋ My Fertility Diary

• Monday

cycle day   basal body temp   vitamin

• Tuesday

cycle day   basal body temp   vitamin

• Wednesday

cycle day   basal body temp   vitamin

• Thursday

cycle day [　]　basal body temp [　]　vitamin [　]

....
....
....

• Friday

cycle day [　]　basal body temp [　]　vitamin [　]

....
....
....

• Saturday

cycle day [　]　basal body temp [　]　vitamin [　]

....
....
....

• Sunday

cycle day [　]　basal body temp [　]　vitamin [　]

....
....
....

My ❀ Thoughts

One thing that always helps us get in the mood is ...

....
....
....
....
....
....
....
....
....
....
....
....

Just ❀ for Dad

You wanted sex every day? Well now you've got it, dad! Results-driven sex may seem strange and pretty unsexy, but you should enjoy all the sex you're having now, because you and mom's sex drives may be different during and immediately after pregnancy. And remember to stay honest with mom about when you're feeling distant, worn out, or like a workhorse.

89

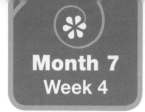

Dress for Romance

Get in the mood for sex and romance by dressing up for your partner. With our hectic schedules, it can be tempting to throw on sweatpants or a ratty T-shirt, but resist the urge, even though it may be comfortable. Instead, wear a dress and jewelry, as you would if you had a date with a new lover. This is especially true for the bedroom! Skip the dowdy nightshirt and wear something more exciting to bed. You will feel sexy, and dad will be turned on by the fact that you took the extra time to look nice.

❋ My Fertility Diary

• Monday

cycle day   basal body temp   vitamin

• Tuesday

cycle day   basal body temp   vitamin

• Wednesday

cycle day   basal body temp   vitamin

• Thursday

cycle day [ ]   basal body temp [ ]   vitamin [ ]

....
....
....

• Friday

cycle day [ ]   basal body temp [ ]   vitamin [ ]

....
....
....

• Saturday

cycle day [ ]   basal body temp [ ]   vitamin [ ]

....
....
....

• Sunday

cycle day [ ]   basal body temp [ ]   vitamin [ ]

....
....
....

My Thoughts

I feel the sexiest when ...

....
....
....
....
....
....
....
....
....
....
....
....
....
....
....

Fertility Lingo

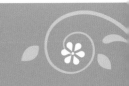

Varicoceles: an abnormal enlargement of the veins in the testes that causes them to drain improperly. Up to 40 percent of men who are infertile have varicoceles, which are thought to affect sperm function by raising the temperature in the testes. Varicoceles can be treated with surgery or minimally invasive vein embolization.

My Reflections

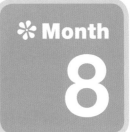

Month

8

"Better keep yourself clean and bright;
you are the window through which
you must see the world."

~ George Bernard Shaw

Kicking the Habit

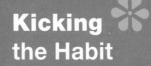

The best way to maximize your chance of conception is to kick your unhealthy habits to the curb, immediately! Not only are these positive lifestyle changes good for you and your partner, but eliminating bad habits will decrease your chance of miscarriage and pregnancy complications. The first few weeks of a pregnancy are the most critical to your baby's development, so if you stop smoking, consuming caffeine, and drinking alcohol and artificial sweeteners now, you will increase your chances of having a quick conception and healthy pregnancy.

Un-Caffeinate

Sorry, but your daily cup of Joe has probably got to go. A study published in the *American Journal of Obstetrics and Gynecology* concluded that women who are actively trying to get pregnant should stop drinking coffee for three months, and hopefully throughout pregnancy. While doctors have varying opinions on the effects of caffeine on fertility and pregnancy, one study found that women who consumed two or more cups of coffee (or five caffeinated sodas) a day had twice the miscarriage risk of women who consumed no caffeine. And don't forget, tea and chocolate also have caffeine in them!

❋ My Fertility Diary

• Monday

cycle day ( ) basal body temp ( ) vitamin ( )

• Tuesday

cycle day ( ) basal body temp ( ) vitamin ( )

• Wednesday

cycle day ( ) basal body temp ( ) vitamin ( )

• Thursday

cycle day ( )   basal body temp ( )   vitamin ( )

....
....
....

• Friday

cycle day ( )   basal body temp ( )   vitamin ( )

....
....
....

• Saturday

cycle day ( )   basal body temp ( )   vitamin ( )

....
....
....

• Sunday

cycle day ( )   basal body temp ( )   vitamin ( )

....
....
....

My Thoughts

List all the caffeinated beverages you drink on a regular basis:

....
....
....
....
....
....
....
....
....
....
....
....

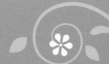

Cockatils to Mocktails

While the jury is still out on the effects of alcohol on fertility, everyone knows that drinking during your pregnancy is a no-go. You may have heard that one glass of wine here and there is fine, but it's smarter to stick to the old adage "better safe than sorry." Therefore, you will probably want to curb alcohol all together while trying to conceive, in preparation for pregnancy. Besides, over-consumption can lead to imbalanced estrogen and progesterone levels, poor eating and sleeping habits, and irregular periods. Try a virgin piña colada at your next happy hour.

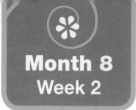

Month 8
Week 2

Say No to Drugs

Think a few puffs of marijuana or recreational use of other illegal drugs won't harm your fertility? Think again. Using illegal drugs, even just occasionally, can disrupt your body's delicate balance and keep you from conceiving. Marijuana, specifically, has been proven to significantly lower fertility in both men and women. Plus, if you do get pregnant, you won't want to have even a small dose of drugs in your system.

❈ My Fertility Diary

• Monday

cycle day ⬚   basal body temp ⬚   vitamin ⬚

• Tuesday

cycle day ⬚   basal body temp ⬚   vitamin ⬚

• Wednesday

cycle day ⬚   basal body temp ⬚   vitamin ⬚

• Thursday

cycle day [ ] basal body temp [ ] vitamin [ ]

....

....

....

• Friday

cycle day [ ] basal body temp [ ] vitamin [ ]

....

....

....

• Saturday

cycle day [ ] basal body temp [ ] vitamin [ ]

....

....

....

• Sunday

cycle day [ ] basal body temp [ ] vitamin [ ]

....

....

....

My ✼ Thoughts

I typically have _____ alcoholic drinks a week, including ...

....

....

....

....

....

....

....

....

....

....

....

....

Quit Smoking, ✼ for Good

You've never had a better reason to stop smoking, for good — your fertility and healthy baby depend on it. This goes for your partner too; secondhand smoke can cause miscarriage, ectopic pregnancy, premature birth, low birth weight, respiratory problems, and Sudden Infant Death Syndrome. If you need extra help quitting smoking, visit www.smokefree.gov for self-help guides, instant support, and interactive tools.

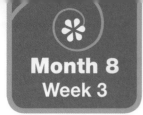

Month 8
Week 3

Your Pregnant Future

Even though you will be the one carrying the baby, your partner should help support you by mirroring your new lifestyle — eating right, exercising, and eliminating unhealthy habits. It's not fair for him to be constantly throwing back cocktails or eating a whole pizza when you're making so many sacrifices for the baby. Plus, it has been shown that men who join their wives in adopting the pregnancy lifestyle report feeling more connected throughout the pregnancy.

❋ My Fertility Diary

• Monday

cycle day ( ) basal body temp ( ) vitamin ( )

....
....
....

• Tuesday

cycle day ( ) basal body temp ( ) vitamin ( )

....
....
....

• Wednesday

cycle day ( ) basal body temp ( ) vitamin ( )

....
....
....

• Thursday

cycle day [ ] basal body temp [ ] vitamin [ ]

....
....
....

• Friday

cycle day [ ] basal body temp [ ] vitamin [ ]

....
....
....

• Saturday

cycle day [ ] basal body temp [ ] vitamin [ ]

....
....
....

• Sunday

cycle day [ ] basal body temp [ ] vitamin [ ]

....
....
....

My ❄ Thoughts

The toughest habit for us to kick will be ...

....
....
....
....
....
....
....
....
....
....
....
....
....
....
....

Fertility ❄ Lingo

Prolactin: elevated levels of this hormone, which can be determined with a blood test, can inhibit ovulation and menstruation. To avoid very high prolactin levels, avoid alcohol, painkillers, marijuana, antidepressant medications, and artificial sweeteners.

Avoid
Artificial Sweeteners

Beware of products that call themselves low-fat, low-sugar, and low-calorie, as they may be full of artificial sweeteners like Aspartame, saccharin, and Splenda. These should be avoided while trying to conceive, because they can affect blood sugar levels and hormonal balance and have been shown to cause infertility and even cancer in rats. To be on the safe side, you'll want to cut back on or cut out things like diet soda for now.

❋ My Fertility Diary

• Monday

cycle day   basal body temp   vitamin

....
....
....

• Tuesday

cycle day   basal body temp   vitamin

....
....
....

• Wednesday

cycle day   basal body temp   vitamin

....
....
....

• Thursday

cycle day [ ] basal body temp [ ] vitamin [ ]

....
....
....

• Friday

cycle day [ ] basal body temp [ ] vitamin [ ]

....
....
....

• Saturday

cycle day [ ] basal body temp [ ] vitamin [ ]

....
....
....

• Sunday

cycle day [ ] basal body temp [ ] vitamin [ ]

....
....
....

My ❋ Thoughts

What healthy habits can we use to replace our bad habits?

....
....
....
....
....
....
....
....
....
....
....
....
....

Questions ❋ for Your Doctor

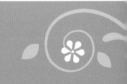

- What amount of caffeine, if any, would you say is safe?
- How many alcoholic drinks should I limit myself to while trying to conceive?
- What is your opinion on consuming artificial sweeteners?
- What can we do if one of us is unable to stop drinking, smoking, or taking drugs?

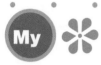

My Reflections

....
....
....
....
....
....
....
....
....
....
....
....
....
....
....
....
....
....
....
....
....
....
....
....

> "Whenever a woman gives birth to a child, she remembers the hard work no more, for the joy that a child has been born into the world."
>
> ~ John 16:21

Stress Less

Trying to conceive can be a very stressful time. Your entire life may seem to revolve around the process, and it is easy to neglect your relationship, friends, and your own needs. While doctors may not totally understand the tie between stress and fertility, countless studies show that chronic stress disrupts the hypothalamus, which oversees hormone production in the thyroid, adrenal glands, ovaries, and testicles. Stress produces the serum cortisol, which can suppress hormones and alter ovulation. The bottom line is this: Stress is linked to disease, anxiety, depression, and irregular menstruation, so nipping stress in the bud during this time is beneficial to conception — as well as your health and sanity!

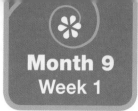

Have a Hobby

Make time each week for a hobby that you find relaxing. For instance, take a pottery or painting class. Join a book club with friends. Or, you might take up a physical hobby, such as golf or tennis. Hobbies have been medically proven to reduce stress and increase happiness. In one study, published in the *Journal of the American Medical Association*, female heart patients reported significant decreases in heart rate and blood pressure while working on a simple craft project. So dive into a hobby that will help de-stress you.

❋ My Fertility Diary

• Monday

cycle day ☐ basal body temp ☐ vitamin ☐

• Tuesday

cycle day ☐ basal body temp ☐ vitamin ☐

• Wednesday

cycle day ☐ basal body temp ☐ vitamin ☐

• Thursday

cycle day ( )   basal body temp ( )   vitamin ( )

....
....
....

• Friday

cycle day ( )   basal body temp ( )   vitamin ( )

....
....
....

• Saturday

cycle day ( )   basal body temp ( )   vitamin ( )

....
....
....

• Sunday

cycle day ( )   basal body temp ( )   vitamin ( )

....
....
....

My Thoughts

The three biggest stressors in my life are ...

....
....
....
....
....
....
....
....
....
....
....
....
....

Did You Know?

In research published in the journal *Human Reproduction*, doctors studying couples trying to conceive found that pregnancy was much more likely to occur during months when couples described themselves as feeling "good, happy, and relaxed." Conception was much less likely to occur during the months when they reported feeling tense, frustrated, or anxious.

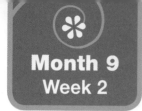

Channel Your Inner Yogini

There's a reason yoga has been around for more than 3,000 years — it strengthens your mind and body. In addition to reducing stress, yoga increases flexibility, stamina and energy; improves balance; and sends oxygen and blood flow to important areas of the body. In a yoga session, you will hold various postures while focusing on breathing, balance, alignment, and different muscle groups. The result is a toned body, less stress, and increased focus. Plus, yoga is one form of exercise that you can maintain all the way through your pregnancy!

❋ My Fertility Diary

• Monday

cycle day ⬚   basal body temp ⬚   vitamin ⬚

....
....
....

• Tuesday

cycle day ⬚   basal body temp ⬚   vitamin ⬚

....
....
....

• Wednesday

cycle day ⬚   basal body temp ⬚   vitamin ⬚

....
....
....

• Thursday

cycle day [ ] basal body temp [ ] vitamin [ ]

....
....
....

• Friday

cycle day [ ] basal body temp [ ] vitamin [ ]

....
....
....

• Saturday

cycle day [ ] basal body temp [ ] vitamin [ ]

....
....
....

• Sunday

cycle day [ ] basal body temp [ ] vitamin [ ]

....
....
....

My Thoughts

My favorite way to de-stress is ...

....
....
....
....
....
....
....
....
....
....
....
....
....

Meditate
to De-Stress

Meditation can be a wonderful stress-relieving exercise. It can be done easily, quickly, inexpensively, and almost anywhere. Meditation instantly calms you by increasing blood flow and slowing the heart rate. According to the National Institutes of Health, just 5 minutes of it can have powerful healing and restorative effects. So find a quiet spot, sit comfortably, and imagine a peaceful place. Take slow, deep breaths. Clear your mind of all stressors. In no time, meditation may become your favorite way to relax!

107

Seek Professional Help with Stress ✣

Because of the stress of trying to conceive, many obstetricians are suggesting that couples have a psychological counseling session. A counselor can offer support and advice if you are having trouble coping or connecting and can provide a forum to discuss feelings and anxieties.

If you are experiencing any of the following issues, you should consider contacting a professional who can help with the stress of this journey:

- Blaming yourself or your partner
- Feelings of losing control
- Guilt over STDs or abortions, which may be affecting conception
- Loss of self-esteem
- Severe mood swings that lead to fighting
- Sexual pressure to perform
- Pressure from family members or friends who know you are trying
- Grief over a miscarriage or false positives
- Anxiety over the possibility of fertility treatments

✣ My Fertility Diary

• Monday

cycle day ⬚   basal body temp ⬚   vitamin ⬚

....
....
....

• Tuesday

cycle day ⬚   basal body temp ⬚   vitamin ⬚

....
....
....

• Wednesday

cycle day ⬚   basal body temp ⬚   vitamin ⬚

....
....
....

• Thursday

cycle day ☐   basal body temp ☐   vitamin ☐

....
....
....

• Friday

cycle day ☐   basal body temp ☐   vitamin ☐

....
....
....

• Saturday

cycle day ☐   basal body temp ☐   vitamin ☐

....
....
....

• Sunday

cycle day ☐   basal body temp ☐   vitamin ☐

....
....
....

My ❋ Thoughts

On a scale of 1 to 10, how stressful is TTC?

....
....
....
....
....
....
....
....
....
....
....
....

Fertility ❋ Lingo

Progesterone and PIBF: progesterone and progesterone-induced blocking factor (PIBF) are both critical to a healthy pregnancy — they prevent the immune system from attacking the placenta and the fetus as foreign objects. Stress has been linked to progesterone suppression.

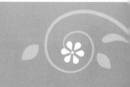

Just for Dad

To ease the constant stress and pressure associated with trying to conceive, plan a TTC-free day for you and your lady. Get out of town, take a bike ride, and have a picnic. Or, make her queen for the day — bring her breakfast in bed, run a hot bath, and give her a foot massage. Create a special day to make time for the two of you — to relax and talk and enjoy each other's company — without a single mention or discussion of trying to conceive. You'll be surprised how even one day off from the process can reinvigorate you.

❀ My Fertility Diary

• Monday

cycle day _____   basal body temp _____   vitamin _____

....
....
....

• Tuesday

cycle day _____   basal body temp _____   vitamin _____

....
....
....

• Wednesday

cycle day _____   basal body temp _____   vitamin _____

....
....
....

• Thursday

cycle day [ ] basal body temp [ ] vitamin [ ]

....
....
....

• Friday

cycle day [ ] basal body temp [ ] vitamin [ ]

....
....
....

• Saturday

cycle day [ ] basal body temp [ ] vitamin [ ]

....
....
....

• Sunday

cycle day [ ] basal body temp [ ] vitamin [ ]

....
....
....

My ✿ Thoughts

One way we can better deal with the stress of TTC is ...

....
....
....
....
....
....
....
....
....
....
....
....
....

Questions ✿ for Your Doctor

Make a list of the top things that stress you and your partner out on a daily or weekly basis. Then, check with your doctor for tips on ways to relax and reduce these stressors.

....
....
....
....

My Reflections

....
....
....
....
....
....
....
....
....
....
....
....
....
....
....
....
....
....
....
....
....
....
....
....
....

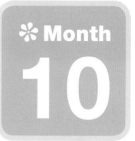

"There are two things in life for which we are never fully prepared, and that is twins."

~ Josh Billings

Our Money, Honey

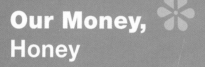

There are countless things to consider when preparing to transition from being a couple to having a family. An important discussion is whether you are financially ready for one! You will soon be paying for a stroller, car seat, baby food, clothes, diapers, a crib, and much more. The Department of Agriculture reports that a child costs about $10,000 a year. You can prepare for pregnancy by discussing the financial details involved with building your family, including health and life insurance, the cost of prenatal care, and more.

Just for Dad

Before mom gets pregnant, you should contact your insurance company to find out exactly what is covered and what your financial responsibilities are when it comes to prenatal and maternity care. Many plans require a flat fee or co-pay of $250 to $500 upon hospital admittance, for example. You will want to know what you're going to owe in advance.

❋ My Fertility Diary

• Monday

cycle day   basal body temp   vitamin

• Tuesday

cycle day   basal body temp   vitamin

• Wednesday

cycle day   basal body temp   vitamin

• Thursday

cycle day [ ] basal body temp [ ] vitamin [ ]

....
....
....

• Friday

cycle day [ ] basal body temp [ ] vitamin [ ]

....
....
....

• Saturday

cycle day [ ] basal body temp [ ] vitamin [ ]

....
....
....

• Sunday

cycle day [ ] basal body temp [ ] vitamin [ ]

....
....
....

My ❋ Thoughts

Some things we save up for ...

....
....
....
....
....
....
....
....
....
....
....
....
....
....

Did You ❋ Know?

The average cost of giving birth to a baby in the United States is more than $8,000, according to a study by the March of Dimes Foundation. Thankfully, due to insurance and government funding, the average out-of-pocket portion is less than $500 per family.

115

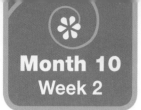

Start Saving Now!

Now is a good time to take a hard look at your finances and come up with a budget you can stick to. Having a baby can be very financially stressful on a marriage if you are not prepared for the associated costs. You can plan to spend between $125,000 and $250,000 until your child turns 18 — and more if you plan to pay for college tuition.

❋ My Fertility Diary

• Monday

cycle day   basal body temp   vitamin

....
....
....

• Tuesday

cycle day   basal body temp   vitamin

....
....
....

• Wednesday

cycle day   basal body temp   vitamin

....
....
....

• Thursday

cycle day [   ]   basal body temp [   ]   vitamin [   ]

....
....
....

• Friday

cycle day [   ]   basal body temp [   ]   vitamin [   ]

....
....
....

• Saturday

cycle day [   ]   basal body temp [   ]   vitamin [   ]

....
....
....

• Sunday

cycle day [   ]   basal body temp [   ]   vitamin [   ]

....
....
....

My ✻ Thoughts

How comfortable are we financially?

....
....
....
....
....
....
....
....
....
....
....
....
....

Look Into ✻ Life Insurance

Most first-time parents purchase "term life insurance." It is the least expensive plan that insures you for a fixed amount at a set premium. As your income increases or your family grows you can increase the amount you are insured. If you already have life insurance, you should reevaluate the beneficiaries specified in your will and choose potential guardians for your child.

Month 10
Week 3

Your Pregnant Future

The most consistent medical costs during pregnancy are the prenatal visits. On average, normal pregnancies require that mom sees her OB-GYN once a month at first and then every one or two weeks until delivery. Depending on your health and the type of insurance you have, pregnancy costs can range from minimal to very expensive. If you have an HMO with a co-pay, these visits shouldn't break the bank. However, some coinsurance plans require up to 30 percent of the cost of each appointment and diagnostic test to be paid by the patient.

My Fertility Diary

• Monday

cycle day | basal body temp | vitamin

• Tuesday

cycle day | basal body temp | vitamin

• Wednesday

cycle day | basal body temp | vitamin

• Thursday

cycle day		basal body temp		vitamin	

....
....
....

• Friday

cycle day		basal body temp		vitamin	

....
....
....

• Saturday

cycle day		basal body temp		vitamin	

....
....
....

• Sunday

cycle day		basal body temp		vitamin	

....
....
....

My ❊

Thoughts

Where will we cut back our spending once we have a baby?

....
....
....
....
....
....
....
....
....
....
....
....
....

Fertility ❊ Lingo

Follicular Phase: the pre-ovulation phase of a woman's cycle during which a new egg is developing within the follicle. This phase is normally between 12 and 14 days.

Consult a Financial Planner

Consult a financial advisor who can help you plan for your growing family. For instance, do you want to start a college fund? Hiring a professional eliminates the stress and confusion that comes with studying market trends and managing your portfolio. Visit the Financial Planning Association online at www.fpanet.org to find a certified financial planner in your area.

☀ My Fertility Diary

• Monday

cycle day ⬜   basal body temp ⬜   vitamin ⬜

....
....
....

• Tuesday

cycle day ⬜   basal body temp ⬜   vitamin ⬜

....
....
....

• Wednesday

cycle day ⬜   basal body temp ⬜   vitamin ⬜

....
....
....

• Thursday

cycle day ⬚   basal body temp ⬚   vitamin ⬚

....
....
....

• Friday

cycle day ⬚   basal body temp ⬚   vitamin ⬚

....
....
....

• Saturday

cycle day ⬚   basal body temp ⬚   vitamin ⬚

....
....
....

• Sunday

cycle day ⬚   basal body temp ⬚   vitamin ⬚

....
....
....

My ✿ Thoughts

Is one of us going to stay home after the baby is born? If yes, will we be comfortable living on one income?

....
....
....
....
....
....
....
....
....
....

Questions ✿ to Ask Yourself

- Do we want to start putting money into a "baby fund" every pay-period?
- Do we need to create a new budget or reevaluate our current one to adjust for the added expense of pregnancy and life with a baby?
- How much will it cost to add a child to our medical insurance policy as an additional dependent?

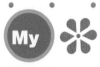

My Reflections

....
....
....
....
....
....
....
....
....
....
....
....
....
....
....
....
....
....
....
....
....
....
....
....

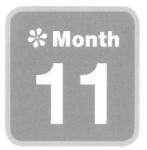

"Wherever you go, go with all your heart."
~ Confucius

Positive Perspective

You've come this far — month 11 — which means while you are more knowledgeable about conception and fertility than ever before, you may be feeling sad or frustrated with your journey. Maintaining a positive perspective when you haven't conceived after months of trying is easier said than done. Forget people who tell you, "Just relax, and you'll get pregnant soon enough." Staying positive means staying tightly connected with your partner, never blaming each other, and being realistic and positive about the future. If you like, you can even start investigating Assisted Reproductive Therapies. Just remember that this journey will all be worth it in the end, when you hold a beautiful baby in your arms!

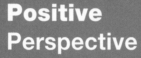

Hop
Online

Need a bit of motivation or an outlet for frustrations? Curious about other couples' fertility journeys? The Internet is a wonderful resource for learning about fertility and pregnancy, as well as finding other people who are going through or have gone through your same experience. There are countless forums and blogs where women and their partners can offer success stories, tips, and support for the tough days. (Just remember to be wary of any medical advice you find online; it's always best to consult your doctor.)

❁ My Fertility Diary

• Monday

cycle day ☐   basal body temp ☐   vitamin ☐

....
....
....

• Tuesday

cycle day ☐   basal body temp ☐   vitamin ☐

....
....
....

• Wednesday

cycle day ☐   basal body temp ☐   vitamin ☐

....
....
....

• Thursday

cycle day ☐ basal body temp ☐ vitamin ☐

....
....
....

• Friday

cycle day ☐ basal body temp ☐ vitamin ☐

....
....
....

• Saturday

cycle day ☐ basal body temp ☐ vitamin ☐

....
....
....

• Sunday

cycle day ☐ basal body temp ☐ vitamin ☐

....
....
....

My ❋
Thoughts

When we need motivation, we remind ourselves ...

....
....
....
....
....
....
....
....
....
....
....
....

Fertility ❋ Lingo

Blocking antibodies: substances created naturally by the body that help fight off bacteria and foreign substances in a woman's immune system to protect the embryo during implantation

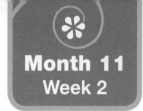

Month 11
Week 2

Pamper
Yourself

Treat yourself to something nice! Be it a new pair of shoes, a facial, or a pedicure, pampering yourself is a way to relax, de-stress, and reward yourself for your diligence in this process. Or, better yet, schedule a couple's massage and unwind together. Some studies have linked the de-stressing qualities of massage to increased fertility.

❋ My Fertility Diary

• Monday

cycle day [   ] basal body temp [   ] vitamin [   ]

....
....
....

• Tuesday

cycle day [   ] basal body temp [   ] vitamin [   ]

....
....
....

• Wednesday

cycle day [   ] basal body temp [   ] vitamin [   ]

....
....
....

126

• Thursday

cycle day ⬚   basal body temp ⬚   vitamin ⬚

....
....
....

• Friday

cycle day ⬚   basal body temp ⬚   vitamin ⬚

....
....
....

• Saturday

cycle day ⬚   basal body temp ⬚   vitamin ⬚

....
....
....

• Sunday

cycle day ⬚   basal body temp ⬚   vitamin ⬚

....
....
....

My ❖ Thoughts

Our favorite way to pamper ourselves is ...

....
....
....
....
....
....
....
....
....
....
....
....
....
....

Avoid ❖ "The Blame Game"

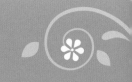

Struggles with conception are no one's fault. It is a common misconception that most couples get pregnant as soon as they start trying, but, in fact, 8 months is the average time it takes. No one is to blame if it takes a little — or a lot — longer. Stay focused and supportive and never point fingers at each other.

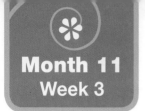

Discuss Your Fertility Future

As you approach a year of TTC, you will want to sit down and have an important conversation: "When do we want to start pursuing other options?" While you may feel disappointed, even angry, the reality is that 90 percent of infertility cases are successfully treated with conventional therapies such as medication or surgery. Decide when will be the best time to actively consider infertility treatments.

❋ My Fertility Diary

• Monday

cycle day   basal body temp   vitamin

• Tuesday

cycle day   basal body temp   vitamin

• Wednesday

cycle day   basal body temp   vitamin

• Thursday

cycle day ⬚   basal body temp ⬚   vitamin ⬚

....
....
....

• Friday

cycle day ⬚   basal body temp ⬚   vitamin ⬚

....
....
....

• Saturday

cycle day ⬚   basal body temp ⬚   vitamin ⬚

....
....
....

• Sunday

cycle day ⬚   basal body temp ⬚   vitamin ⬚

....
....
....

My ❋

Thoughts

When we feel anxious or frustrated, we find that it helps to ...

....
....
....
....
....
....
....
....
....
....

Did You ❋ Know?

Since the American Society for Reproductive Medicine began counting in 1985, almost 500,000 babies have been born in the United States as a result of Assisted Reproductive Technology (ART). Approximately one in every hundred babies born in the United States is conceived using ART.

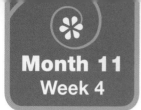

Guilt-Free
Fertility

In the same sense that you should never place blame on each other, you should never feel guilty for not getting pregnant. Never allow yourself to think "I should have relaxed more," "I should never have had that drink," or, "If only I hadn't had that abortion." Infertility is not a punishment — it is a medical problem with many avenues for managing it. Lean on each other. Talk it out when you are scared or sad. And remember that every couple's conception journey takes a different path.

❊ My Fertility Diary

• Monday

cycle day ⬭   basal body temp ⬭   vitamin ⬭

....
....
....

• Tuesday

cycle day ⬭   basal body temp ⬭   vitamin ⬭

....
....
....

• Wednesday

cycle day ⬭   basal body temp ⬭   vitamin ⬭

....
....
....

• Thursday

cycle day [ ]   basal body temp [ ]   vitamin [ ]

....
....
....

• Friday

cycle day [ ]   basal body temp [ ]   vitamin [ ]

....
....
....

• Saturday

cycle day [ ]   basal body temp [ ]   vitamin [ ]

....
....
....

• Sunday

cycle day [ ]   basal body temp [ ]   vitamin [ ]

....
....
....

My ❋ Thoughts

We support each other by ...

....
....
....
....
....
....
....
....
....
....
....
....
....
....
....

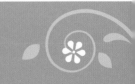

Questions ❋ for Your Doctor

- What else can I change or adjust that may affect our chances for conception?
- Are there supplemental therapies you support that may boost fertility, such as acupuncture or massage?
- Should we consider other tests to evaluate our fertility?

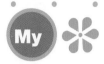

My Reflections

....
....
....
....
....
....
....
....
....
....
....
....
....
....
....
....
....
....
....
....
....
....

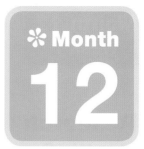

"Babies are such a nice way to start people."

~ Don Herold

A Pregnancy Preview

Although your conception journey is still underway, it is a good idea to start thinking about the effects having a baby will have on your life. When your family goes from two to three or more, everything will change — from your social life to your career to your relationship. There will be much to consider, such as maternity and paternity leave, choosing a health care provider, and much more. Start thinking ahead now because you will be overwhelmed once pregnancy hits!

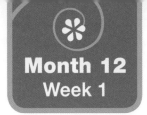

Month 12
Week 1

Research
Health Care Providers

Your first prenatal exam will be when you are about 8 weeks pregnant, so you should start researching health care providers now. You can stick with the OB-GYN or midwife who has overseen your regular gynecological care, although not all OB-GYNs specialize in female reproductive health and pregnancy. Or, you may want to find an obstetrician, who is trained to perform more difficult vaginal births and cesarean sections, as well as manage pregnancies with any complications.

❋ My Fertility Diary

• Monday

cycle day ⬭   basal body temp ⬭   vitamin ⬭

....
....
....

• Tuesday

cycle day ⬭   basal body temp ⬭   vitamin ⬭

....
....
....

• Wednesday

cycle day ⬭   basal body temp ⬭   vitamin ⬭

....
....
....

• Thursday

cycle day ⬚ basal body temp ⬚ vitamin ⬚

....
....
....

• Friday

cycle day ⬚ basal body temp ⬚ vitamin ⬚

....
....
....

• Saturday

cycle day ⬚ basal body temp ⬚ vitamin ⬚

....
....
....

• Sunday

cycle day ⬚ basal body temp ⬚ vitamin ⬚

....
....
....

My ✿ Thoughts

What are we most looking forward to about pregnancy?

....
....
....
....
....
....
....
....
....
....
....

Maternity & ✿ Paternity Leave

The Family Medical Leave Act (FMLA) provides employees with up to 12 weeks of unpaid leave any time during the first 12 months after the birth or adoption of a child, with the right to return to their same salary, title, and benefits. FMLA leave can be taken before birth for prenatal care, health issues, or preparing for the baby. Check with your employers to determine how they require you to request and take maternity or paternity leave.

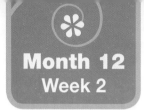

Month 12
Week 2

Just for Dad

Do you host a poker game at your house every week? Is happy hour with friends a typical Friday night? Your social life will need to shift with pregnancy. Your pregnant partner will need to stay away from alcohol, cigarettes, and secondhand smoke. Additionally, pregnancy can be draining and will probably mean your sweetheart is ready for bed earlier than normal. This is an important time to bond with mom and acknowledge that a weekly guys' night out may not be in the cards for a while.

❋ My Fertility Diary

• Monday

cycle day | basal body temp | vitamin

• Tuesday

cycle day | basal body temp | vitamin

• Wednesday

cycle day | basal body temp | vitamin

• Thursday

cycle day [ ]   basal body temp [ ]   vitamin [ ]

....
....
....

• Friday

cycle day [ ]   basal body temp [ ]   vitamin [ ]

....
....
....

• Saturday

cycle day [ ]   basal body temp [ ]   vitamin [ ]

....
....
....

• Sunday

cycle day [ ]   basal body temp [ ]   vitamin [ ]

....
....
....

My ❁ Thoughts

The biggest way we anticipate our lives will change with pregnancy is ...

....
....
....
....
....
....
....
....
....
....
....
....

Did You ❁ Know?

Some women report knowing that they were pregnant even before their missed period solely because of tenderness, soreness, or swelling of the breasts and nipples. This is often the very first symptom of pregnancy.

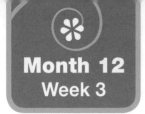

Month 12
Week 3

Your Pregnant Future

During pregnancy, your libido may not always match dad's — especially in the first few months when morning sickness and fatigue take their toll. Adding to the confusion, the hormones surging through your body can make a loving caress feel like sandpaper one minute, while the same touch a few hours later may lead to some of the hottest sex of your life. Good thing you practiced patience and communication during your conception journey!

❀ My Fertility Diary

• Monday

cycle day ⬚ basal body temp ⬚ vitamin ⬚

....
....
....

• Tuesday

cycle day ⬚ basal body temp ⬚ vitamin ⬚

....
....
....

• Wednesday

cycle day ⬚ basal body temp ⬚ vitamin ⬚

....
....
....

• Thursday

cycle day ☐ basal body temp ☐ vitamin ☐

....
....
....

• Friday

cycle day ☐ basal body temp ☐ vitamin ☐

....
....
....

• Saturday

cycle day ☐ basal body temp ☐ vitamin ☐

....
....
....

• Sunday

cycle day ☐ basal body temp ☐ vitamin ☐

....
....
....

My ✿
Thoughts

**Pregnancy is a/n ....
thought for me
...** ....
....
....
....
....
....
....
....
....
....
....
....

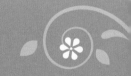

Fertility ✿ Lingo

Implantation: the moment a fertilized egg attaches itself to the uterine wall, resulting in a pregnancy. Implantation may occur between 5 and 10 days after ovulation.

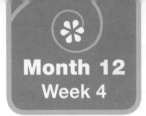

Staying Home with Baby

Do you plan to be a stay-at-home mom or a working mother with a career? Truly, you will want to experience what it is like to be home with a baby before making this important choice. Many mothers who decided they would not return to work after having a baby find they do not enjoy the confines of staying at home. Still, other women find they have no interest in returning to their jobs once they get a chance to be a mom.

✽ **My Fertility Diary**

• **Monday**

cycle day   basal body temp   vitamin

• **Tuesday**

cycle day   basal body temp   vitamin

• **Wednesday**

cycle day   basal body temp   vitamin

• Thursday

cycle day [   ]   basal body temp [   ]   vitamin [   ]

....
....
....

• Friday

cycle day [   ]   basal body temp [   ]   vitamin [   ]

....
....
....

• Saturday

cycle day [   ]   basal body temp [   ]   vitamin [   ]

....
....
....

• Sunday

cycle day [   ]   basal body temp [   ]   vitamin [   ]

....
....
....

My �֎ Thoughts

Our conception journey, thus far, has been ...

....
....
....
....
....
....
....
....
....
....
....
....
....

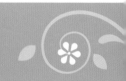

Questions ✖ for Your Doctor

- Am I at risk for pregnancy complications?
- How can I minimize the risk of complications?
- Are there any lifestyle changes I still need to make?

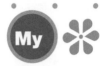

My Reflections

....
....
....
....
....
....
....
....
....
....
....
....
....
....
....
....
....
....
....
....
....
....

When It Takes
a Little Longer

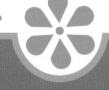

So, you've been filling out this fertility journal for 12 months and still no luck getting pregnant. Actually, conception has very little to do with luck, and much more to do with age and various medical factors. And while you may feel like everyone around you is getting pregnant and having babies, the fact is, 6.1 million Americans — about 10 percent of the reproductive-age population — experience infertility. The good news is that there is usually a treatable reason for delayed conception, and true sterility is actually quite rare.

In women under 35, infertility is defined as the failure to conceive after one year of intercourse without using contraceptives. For women older than 35, this timeframe shortens to six months. Pregnancy rates begin to decline in the early 30s, with the most significant decline in the mid-30s. About 10 percent of women under 35, and 22 percent of women ages 35 to 39, deal with infertility. Once you reach age 40, those who experience infertility nearly triples to 29 percent.

In need of some good news? About 90 percent of couples dealing with infertility are treated with low-tech options like fertility drugs or noninvasive surgeries.

The first thing to remember when you are dealing with infertility is that it is no one's fault. While infertility was historically thought of as a female issue, we now know that men and women contribute equally to fertility problems. According to the American Society for Reproductive Medicine, infertility is a female problem in 35 percent of cases, a male problem in 35 percent of cases, a combined problem of the couple in 20 percent of cases, and unexplained in 10 percent of cases. Therefore, when you schedule a visit with a fertility specialist to diagnose your hold-up, it is essential that both you and your partner be evaluated.

No matter what your diagnosis, the good news is that about 90 percent of couples dealing with infertility are treated with low-tech options like fertility drugs or noninvasive surgeries, with less than 3 percent needing Assisted Reproductive Technologies (ART) like IVF. And of those treated for infertility, nearly 70 percent will go on to have a baby.

Causes of Infertility

The first step is consulting a fertility specialist who can administer an infertility evaluation for you and your partner. Dad will have a sperm analysis, which will examine sperm count, motility, size and shape of the sperm, velocity, and volume.

> Nearly 500,000 babies have been born in the U.S. as a result of Assisted Reproductive Technology since 1985.

You will have a complete evaluation to determine any abnormalities, including a cervical exam, blood test, pelvic ultrasound, X-ray of the fallopian tubes, and post-coital cervical mucus test. Remember to bring this journal with you to your appointment, because your doctor may be able to find important clues by reviewing your charted ovulation cycle.

 The following are the most common diagnoses for both men and women:

Ovulatory Dysfunction

Oligovulation and anovulation are types of ovulatory dysfunction in which a woman will have either irregular ovulation or completely absent ovulation. Naturally, it is difficult or impossible to conceive when ovulation is very sporadic or if no egg present. Also, if the length of your cycle varies widely from month to month, making it difficult to track your ovulation, this may be considered a form of ovulatory dysfunction. You may have a clue that this is your problem just from charting your cycle all these months.

Ovulatory dysfunction affects 40 percent of women facing infertility and is usually treatable with lifestyle changes or fertility medications, such as Clomid.

Tubal Blockage

The fallopian tubes, which carry the egg from the ovaries to the uterus to be implanted, can become blocked on one or both sides. Sometimes, a partial blockage can lead to tubal or ectopic pregnancy. The most common cause of blocked fallopian tubes is scarring and adhesions from pelvic inflammatory disease (PID), which is most often caused by a past or current STD. Past miscarriages or abortions can also cause scarring and tubal blockage.

IVF, or in vitro fertilization, was first introduced in 1978 and now accounts for more than 99 percent of Assisted Reproductive Technologies.

Endometriosis is another cause of tubal blockage, characterized by painful menstruation. With this condition, the tissue necessary for implantation, which normally lines only the uterus, grows abnormally in the fallopian tubes or other reproductive organs, causing blockage.

Men can also experience tubal blockage in the vas deferens or epididymis, which prevent the sperm from traveling to meet the egg. Many times, this is the result of STDs such as chlamydia or gonorrhea.

Your doctor will test for tubal blockage with an ultrasound or special X-ray, called a hysterosalpingogram (HSG). If blocked fallopian tubes are determined to be the cause of your infertility, as is the case with 40 percent of infertile women, you may need laparoscopic surgery to remove the adhesions and blockage. Surgery can also repair blockages in men. In more severe cases, you will skip surgery and go straight to IVF treatments.

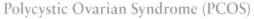

Polycystic Ovarian Syndrome (PCOS)

Polycystic ovarian syndrome (PCOS) is a common cause of infertility in women that can lead to ovulatory dysfunction, cystic ovaries, or miscarriage. PCOS is a hormonal disorder that is most often associated with an absent or irregular period or a cycle that lasts more than 40 days. Additionally, women with PCOS may have problems with acne, abnormal hair growth, obesity, and diabetes.

Diagnosis of PCOS requires blood testing for a variety of hormones. Treatment often includes lifestyle changes, such as weight loss, as well as fertility drugs.

Varicoceles

Varicoceles affect men only and are characterized as an abnormal enlargement of the veins in the testes that causes them to drain improperly. While the effects aren't completely understood, it is thought that varicoceles hurt sperm function by raising the temperature in the testes.

> Although less than 10 percent of couples choose to go this route, the live birth rate for egg and/or sperm donation is between 40 and 45 percent.

Up 40 percent of men who are infertile have varicoceles, although they usually go unnoticed until infertility becomes an issue. They can be treated with surgery or a minimally invasive vein embolization.

Treatments & Procedures

As we mentioned, up to 90 percent of couples experiencing infertility can be treated with medications or surgery, so those will be the first routes your fertility specialist or reproductive endocrinologist will take.

Fertility Drugs

Fertility medications come in oral and injectible forms and can be coupled with IVF, if you end up utilizing that type of treatment down the line. Multiples — twins, triplets, or more — are not unusual when using fertility drugs. Common fertility drugs include:

• **Clomiphene Citrate:** Most commonly known as Clomid (or Serophene), this oral tablet is generally the first drug used in treatment to stimulate ovulation in women with irregular cycles. In addition to being fairly inexpensive, another perk of Clomid is that it is only taken for a few days during each cycle.

• **Follicle Stimulating Hormone (FSH):** An injection given below the skin mimics naturally produced FSH, which stimulates follicle growth in the ovaries and the release of eggs.

• **Synthetic Human Chorionic Gonadotropin (hCG):** These intramuscular injections are used to induce the release of the egg from the follicle. Ovulation usually occurs approximately 36 hours after injection. In men, hCG can encourage the testes to produce testosterone.

• **Human Menopausal Gonadotropins (hMG):** The most potent ovulation medication used today, this injectible drug contains FSH and LH (luteinizing hormone) to encourage the ovaries to produce multiple eggs. It can also be used in men to induce sperm production.

Surgical Procedures

In many infertility patients, a simple surgical procedure can right blockages or other issues standing in the way of conception. Here are some of the common procedures:

• **Laparoscopic surgery:** This minor surgical procedure is actually also a diagnostic test; if problems are found during the test they can be surgically repaired at that time. The minimally invasive surgery involves inserting a laparoscope in through a small incision in the navel so the doctor can view the reproductive organs. Laparoscopic surgery can treat blockages, adhesions, endometriosis, ovarian cysts, fibroids, or ectopic pregnancy.

• **Tubal surgery:** In 35 percent of female infertility patients, the hysterosalpingogram (HSG) X-ray finds blockages or adhesions in the fallopian tubes or problems with the lining of other areas in the pelvis. Laparoscopic surgery can be done to open fallopian tubes, reconnect them, or remove scar tissue. This procedure is mainly done on women younger than 35, and success rates are good.

• **Varicocelectomy:** This minor surgery is done on men with varicoceles, or varicose veins that inhibit sperm production. A surgeon makes a small incision in the abdomen and repairs the veins, thereby increasing blood flow and reducing the body temperature in the scrotum. This procedure may normalize sperm production.

• **Vasovasostomy:** Done on an outpatient basis under local or general anesthesia, this surgery repairs blockages in the vas deferens and epididymis.

Assisted Reproductive Technology (ART)

Sometimes, fertility medications alone are not successful or blockages and scarring are not surgically repairable. In this case, Assisted Reproductive Technology (ART) is the next step.

Historically, ART has referred to infertility therapies that boost the chances of conception, including IUI, ICSI, IVF, GIFT, and ZIFT. These days, ART has come to represent procedures that involve the handling of eggs or embryos — specifically in vitro fertilization (IVF), which is the most popular form of treatment. (While this section will help you become familiar with several forms of ART, IVF will be the most relevant for most couples. The upcoming chapter will deal solely with tracking your IVF cycles.)

ART can also be performed using donor eggs and/or sperm. Although less than 10 percent of couples choose to go this route, the live birth rate for egg and/or sperm donation is between 40 and 45 percent. For older women who generally produce eggs that are of lower quality, donor eggs may be the best option.

• **IUI (intrauterine insemination):** IUI involves injecting specially washed sperm directly into the uterus during ovulation. IUI may be used in cases of unexplained infertility, hostile cervical mucus, or male sperm abnormalities. IUI may also be performed with donor sperm. Success depends on the availability of high-quality eggs. The advantage of IUI is the cost, which is much lower than IVF.

• **ICSI (intracytoplasmic sperm injection):** ICSI is often used if sperm analysis detects severe male infertility. It involves injecting a single sperm directly into the egg and is often used to complement IVF treatments.

• **GIFT (gamete intrafallopian transfer) & ZIFT (zygote intrafallopian transfer):** GIFT involves placing the unfertilized egg and sperm, or gametes, into the fallopian tubes, where nature goes to work. This is only for women who have at least one unblocked fallopian tube.

 With ZIFT, the egg and sperm are fertilized outside the body in a laboratory, and the zygote is placed into one of the fallopian tubes, usually with laparoscopic surgery.

• **IVF (in vitro fertilization):** IVF is the most common ART therapy and currently accounts for more than 99 percent of ART procedures. IVF was introduced in 1978, when Louise Brown was born as a result of IVF in Great Britain — deemed the first "test-tube" baby. It is best for women with blocked fallopian tubes or cases in which men have low sperm count.

IVF is a multi-step process that begins when fertility drugs are given to promote multiple egg production during ovulation. The eggs are then retrieved through minor surgery and combined with sperm and special nutrients in a lab dish. (In women over 40, donor eggs are generally used.) Once fertilization occurs and the eggs and sperm are cultured into early embryos, the embryos are surgically implanted into the woman's uterus. A pregnancy test is performed after 14 days — thus, the term Two-Week Wait — to see if the embryo transfer (ET) was a success.

According to The Centers for Disease Control, the live birth rate per transfer for IVF is 34 percent. The likelihood of multiple pregnancies is high, since several embryos may be implanted at one time.

While IVF may be the saving grace for couples experiencing infertility, the downside is that each cycle is very expensive and more than one cycle is often necessary. The average cost of an IVF cycle in the United States is $12,400, but each cycle can cost as much as $25,000.

Insurance Coverage for ART

Assisted Reproductive Technologies, especially IVF, can very expensive. Unfortunately, not all insurance plans and states provide coverage. The American Society for Reproductive Medicine reports that only 14 states (Arkansas, California, Connecticut, Hawaii, Illinois, Maryland, Massachusetts, Montana, New Jersey, New York, Ohio, Rhode Island, Texas and West Virginia) currently have laws that require insurance companies to cover all or part of infertility diagnosis and treatment. In addition, the laws vary greatly from state to state.

It is best to research your state's policies and call your insurance provider to determine what is and is not covered before beginning treatment. Another great resource is RESOLVE (www.resolve.org), a non-profit organization whose mission is to provide advocacy, support, and information to people who are experiencing infertility and increase public awareness of infertility issues.

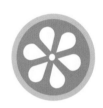

Fertility
Treatment Journal

Charting Your Fertility Treatments

Now that you've decided to pursue IVF, you will need the second portion of this journal, in which you will chart your fertility treatments. It now becomes very important to chart your fertility medications, appointments, and instructions from your doctor. Many of these medications have specific instructions about how and when to take them, so it is important to write down the name, time, and dosage you take of each medication.

This section of the journal has space to document two cycles of IVF, with six weeks in each cycle. The first two weeks will entail taking medications like Gonadotropin Releasing Hormone Analogues (GnRH-a), which will suppress your cycle.

Next, you will spend weeks three and four documenting hormone injections of medications you will take to stimulate ovulation (such as hCG). An ultrasound will confirm that the eggs are ready to be retrieved and fertilized in the laboratory. The fertilized eggs will sit in a special cocktail of nutrients for three to five days before being implanted into the uterus. You will be asked to refrain from most physical activity for the next 48 hours.

Finally, weeks five and six comprise the Two-Week Wait. This means that about two weeks after egg retrieval, you will take a pregnancy test to see if any of the embryos implanted successfully.

The Dreaded Two-Week Wait

In the classic children's book *Charlotte's Web*, author E.B. White writes, "Life is always a rich and steady time when you are waiting for something to happen or to hatch." Unfortunately, this isn't true for couples who have spent many months trying to conceive and have now turned to IVF. The 14 days between embryo transfer and the pregnancy test are often filled with anxiety and worry — this is what is called the Two-Week Wait (TWW), and it is the time that couples going through IVF most dread.

You and your partner will go through a huge range of emotions during the TWW — everything from panic to exhilaration to obsession. In fact, many women become completely consumed with spotting signs that pregnancy has hit during the TWW — "Do I feel nauseous? Do my breasts feel sore?" The reality is, many of these symptoms are a result of the fertility drugs you are taking, so don't jump to any conclusions. The only thing you can really trust is the test at the end of the TWW.

There are countless ways to avoid making yourselves crazy, from taking a walk to finding a hobby to simply sitting down together and talking about how you're feeling. And, if you find that there are emotions you are afraid to express out loud, try keeping a journal. This book offers you space at the end of each treatment cycle to write down your thoughts, worries, and daydreams.

And, perhaps the best way to stay calm and positive during the dreaded TWW is to remind each other of the saying, "Grant me the serenity to accept the things I cannot change." Stressing and obsessing for two weeks won't help you get pregnant. Stay busy, and focus on anticipating the joy you will feel when you do get that positive pregnancy test.

Journaling After Each Cycle

You have been given two full cycles in this section, with pages at the end of each cycle to journal. There, you will find space to vent, where you can write down your hopes and joys, as well as your worries while you sit tight throughout the TWW. Come up with ways you can stay busy and pass the time. Think of ways you can pamper yourself and dad after several difficult weeks of IVF treatments.

You should also practice staying positive by replacing negative thoughts with positive ones. For instance, if you find yourself thinking, "It won't work; I will never get pregnant," write down a series of positive statements to replace that thought. Come up with statements like, "We have done everything in our power to have a baby." And, remember to be grateful for the things you do have in your life, which are surely plentiful.

> "Faith makes all things possible... love makes all things easy."
> ~ Dwight Moody

Finally, you can maintain your perspective and motivation by filling out the section that describes why this process is worth the wait. Write about why you and your partner are so excited to have a baby and a family. Why do you know you will make good parents? What are the personality and physical traits you both hope to pass on? You may even feel inclined to write a letter to your future child. When you eventually hold a child in your arms — whether it is sooner, or whether it's later — you will know instantly that all your hard work was worth it.

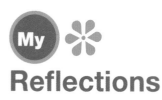

Reflections

....
....
....
....
....
....
....
....
....
....
....
....
....
....
....
....
....
....
....
....
....
....
....
....

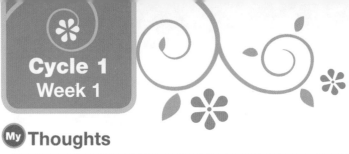

Cycle 1
Week 1

My Thoughts

....
....
....

❈ Date .... cycle day ⬭ vitamin ⬭ test results ....

Doctor's Instructions:

....

....

....

....

....

....

Medications:

Oral	Inj.	Time	Name	Qty.
☐	☐	....	....	....
☐	☐	....	....	....
☐	☐	....	....	....
☐	☐	....	....	....
☐	☐	....	....	....

❈ Date .... cycle day ⬭ vitamin ⬭ test results ....

Doctor's Instructions:

....

....

....

....

....

....

Medications:

Oral	Inj.	Time	Name	Qty.
☐	☐	....	....	....
☐	☐	....	....	....
☐	☐	....	....	....
☐	☐	....	....	....
☐	☐	....	....	....

❈ Date .... cycle day ⬭ vitamin ⬭ test results ....

Doctor's Instructions:

....

....

....

....

....

....

Medications:

Oral	Inj.	Time	Name	Qty.
☐	☐	....	....	....
☐	☐	....	....	....
☐	☐	....	....	....
☐	☐	....	....	....
☐	☐	....	....	....

✿ Date .... cycle day [ ] vitamin [ ] test results ....

Doctor's Instructions:

....
....
....
....
....
....

Medications:

Oral	Inj.	Time	Name	Qty.
[ ]	[ ]	....	....	......
[ ]	[ ]	....	....	......
[ ]	[ ]	....	....	......
[ ]	[ ]	....	....	......
[ ]	[ ]	....	....	......

✿ Date .... cycle day [ ] vitamin [ ] test results ....

Doctor's Instructions:

....
....
....
....
....
....

Medications:

Oral	Inj.	Time	Name	Qty.
[ ]	[ ]	....	....	......
[ ]	[ ]	....	....	......
[ ]	[ ]	....	....	......
[ ]	[ ]	....	....	......
[ ]	[ ]	....	....	......

✿ Date .... cycle day [ ] vitamin [ ] test results ....

Doctor's Instructions:

....
....
....
....
....
....

Medications:

Oral	Inj.	Time	Name	Qty.
[ ]	[ ]	....	....	......
[ ]	[ ]	....	....	......
[ ]	[ ]	....	....	......
[ ]	[ ]	....	....	......
[ ]	[ ]	....	....	......

✿ Date .... cycle day [ ] vitamin [ ] test results ....

Doctor's Instructions:

....
....
....
....
....
....

Medications:

Oral	Inj.	Time	Name	Qty.
[ ]	[ ]	....	....	......
[ ]	[ ]	....	....	......
[ ]	[ ]	....	....	......
[ ]	[ ]	....	....	......
[ ]	[ ]	....	....	......

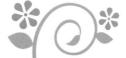

Cycle 1
Week 2

My Thoughts

....

....

....

Date .... cycle day ▢ vitamin ▢ test results ....

Doctor's Instructions:

....

....

....

....

....

....

Medications:

Oral	Inj.	Time	Name	Qty.
▢	▢	....	....	....
▢	▢	....	....	....
▢	▢	....	....	....
▢	▢	....	....	....
▢	▢	....	....	....

Date .... cycle day ▢ vitamin ▢ test results ....

Doctor's Instructions:

....

....

....

....

....

....

Medications:

Oral	Inj.	Time	Name	Qty.
▢	▢	....	....	....
▢	▢	....	....	....
▢	▢	....	....	....
▢	▢	....	....	....
▢	▢	....	....	....

Date .... cycle day ▢ vitamin ▢ test results ....

Doctor's Instructions:

....

....

....

....

....

....

Medications:

Oral	Inj.	Time	Name	Qty.
▢	▢	....	....	....
▢	▢	....	....	....
▢	▢	....	....	....
▢	▢	....	....	....
▢	▢	....	....	....

❋ Date .... cycle day [ ] vitamin [ ] test results ....

Doctor's Instructions:

....

....

....

....

....

....

Medications:

Oral	Inj.	Time	Name	Qty.
[ ]	[ ]	....	....	....
[ ]	[ ]	....	....	....
[ ]	[ ]	....	....	....
[ ]	[ ]	....	....	....
[ ]	[ ]	....	....	....

❋ Date .... cycle day [ ] vitamin [ ] test results ....

Doctor's Instructions:

....

....

....

....

....

....

Medications:

Oral	Inj.	Time	Name	Qty.
[ ]	[ ]	....	....	....
[ ]	[ ]	....	....	....
[ ]	[ ]	....	....	....
[ ]	[ ]	....	....	....
[ ]	[ ]	....	....	....

❋ Date .... cycle day [ ] vitamin [ ] test results ....

Doctor's Instructions:

....

....

....

....

....

....

Medications:

Oral	Inj.	Time	Name	Qty.
[ ]	[ ]	....	....	....
[ ]	[ ]	....	....	....
[ ]	[ ]	....	....	....
[ ]	[ ]	....	....	....
[ ]	[ ]	....	....	....

❋ Date .... cycle day [ ] vitamin [ ] test results ....

Doctor's Instructions:

....

....

....

....

....

....

Medications:

Oral	Inj.	Time	Name	Qty.
[ ]	[ ]	....	....	....
[ ]	[ ]	....	....	....
[ ]	[ ]	....	....	....
[ ]	[ ]	....	....	....
[ ]	[ ]	....	....	....

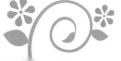

Cycle 1
Week 3

My Thoughts

....

....

....

※ **Date** .... cycle day ◯ vitamin ◯ test results ....

Doctor's Instructions:

....

....

....

....

....

....

Medications:

Oral	Inj.	Time	Name	Qty.
◻	◻			
◻	◻			
◻	◻			
◻	◻			
◻	◻			

※ **Date** .... cycle day ◯ vitamin ◯ test results ....

Doctor's Instructions:

....

....

....

....

....

....

Medications:

Oral	Inj.	Time	Name	Qty.
◻	◻			
◻	◻			
◻	◻			
◻	◻			
◻	◻			

※ **Date** .... cycle day ◯ vitamin ◯ test results ....

Doctor's Instructions:

....

....

....

....

....

....

Medications:

Oral	Inj.	Time	Name	Qty.
◻	◻			
◻	◻			
◻	◻			
◻	◻			
◻	◻			

❊ Date .... cycle day ▢ vitamin ▢ test results ....

Doctor's Instructions:

....
....
....
....
....
....

Medications:

Oral	Inj.	Time	Name	Qty.
▢	▢	....	....	....
▢	▢	....	....	....
▢	▢	....	....	....
▢	▢	....	....	....
▢	▢	....	....	....

❊ Date .... cycle day ▢ vitamin ▢ test results ....

Doctor's Instructions:

....
....
....
....
....
....

Medications:

Oral	Inj.	Time	Name	Qty.
▢	▢	....	....	....
▢	▢	....	....	....
▢	▢	....	....	....
▢	▢	....	....	....
▢	▢	....	....	....

❊ Date .... cycle day ▢ vitamin ▢ test results ....

Doctor's Instructions:

....
....
....
....
....
....

Medications:

Oral	Inj.	Time	Name	Qty.
▢	▢	....	....	....
▢	▢	....	....	....
▢	▢	....	....	....
▢	▢	....	....	....
▢	▢	....	....	....

❊ Date .... cycle day ▢ vitamin ▢ test results ....

Doctor's Instructions:

....
....
....
....
....
....

Medications:

Oral	Inj.	Time	Name	Qty.
▢	▢	....	....	....
▢	▢	....	....	....
▢	▢	....	....	....
▢	▢	....	....	....
▢	▢	....	....	....

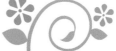

Cycle 1
Week 4

My Thoughts

....
....
....

✱ Date .... cycle day ▢ vitamin ▢ test results ....

Doctor's Instructions:

....
....
....
....
....
....

Medications:

Oral	Inj.	Time	Name	Qty.
▢	▢	....	....	....
▢	▢	....	....	....
▢	▢	....	....	....
▢	▢	....	....	....
▢	▢	....	....	....

✱ Date .... cycle day ▢ vitamin ▢ test results ....

Doctor's Instructions:

....
....
....
....
....
....

Medications:

Oral	Inj.	Time	Name	Qty.
▢	▢	....	....	....
▢	▢	....	....	....
▢	▢	....	....	....
▢	▢	....	....	....
▢	▢	....	....	....

✱ Date .... cycle day ▢ vitamin ▢ test results ....

Doctor's Instructions:

....
....
....
....
....
....

Medications:

Oral	Inj.	Time	Name	Qty.
▢	▢	....	....	....
▢	▢	....	....	....
▢	▢	....	....	....
▢	▢	....	....	....
▢	▢	....	....	....

✿ Date .... cycle day ▢ vitamin ▢ test results ....

Doctor's Instructions:

Medications:

Oral	Inj.	Time	Name	Qty.
▢	▢	....	....	....
▢	▢	....	....	....
▢	▢	....	....	....
▢	▢	....	....	....
▢	▢	....	....	....
▢	▢	....	....	....

....
....
....
....
....
....
....

✿ Date .... cycle day ▢ vitamin ▢ test results ....

Doctor's Instructions:

Medications:

Oral	Inj.	Time	Name	Qty.
▢	▢	....	....	....
▢	▢	....	....	....
▢	▢	....	....	....
▢	▢	....	....	....
▢	▢	....	....	....
▢	▢	....	....	....

....
....
....
....
....
....

✿ Date .... cycle day ▢ vitamin ▢ test results ....

Doctor's Instructions:

Medications:

Oral	Inj.	Time	Name	Qty.
▢	▢	....	....	....
▢	▢	....	....	....
▢	▢	....	....	....
▢	▢	....	....	....
▢	▢	....	....	....
▢	▢	....	....	....

....
....
....
....
....
....

✿ Date .... cycle day ▢ vitamin ▢ test results ....

Doctor's Instructions:

Medications:

Oral	Inj.	Time	Name	Qty.
▢	▢	....	....	....
▢	▢	....	....	....
▢	▢	....	....	....
▢	▢	....	....	....
▢	▢	....	....	....
▢	▢	....	....	....

....
....
....
....
....
....

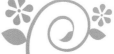

165

Cycle 1
Week 5

My Thoughts

....
....
....
....

Date .... cycle day ⬜ vitamin ⬜ test results ....

Doctor's Instructions:

....
....
....
....
....
....

Medications:

Oral	Inj.	Time	Name	Qty.
⬜	⬜	....	....	....
⬜	⬜	....	....	....
⬜	⬜	....	....	....
⬜	⬜	....	....	....
⬜	⬜	....	....	....

Date .... cycle day ⬜ vitamin ⬜ test results ....

Doctor's Instructions:

....
....
....
....
....
....

Medications:

Oral	Inj.	Time	Name	Qty.
⬜	⬜	....	....	....
⬜	⬜	....	....	....
⬜	⬜	....	....	....
⬜	⬜	....	....	....
⬜	⬜	....	....	....

Date .... cycle day ⬜ vitamin ⬜ test results ....

Doctor's Instructions:

....
....
....
....
....
....

Medications:

Oral	Inj.	Time	Name	Qty.
⬜	⬜	....	....	....
⬜	⬜	....	....	....
⬜	⬜	....	....	....
⬜	⬜	....	....	....
⬜	⬜	....	....	....

❊ Date .... cycle day ⬭ vitamin ⬭ test results ....

Doctor's Instructions:

....

....

....

....

....

....

....

Medications:

Oral	Inj.	Time	Name	Qty.
☐	☐	....	....	....
☐	☐	....	....	....
☐	☐	....	....	....
☐	☐	....	....	....
☐	☐	....	....	....

❊ Date .... cycle day ⬭ vitamin ⬭ test results ....

Doctor's Instructions:

....

....

....

....

....

....

....

Medications:

Oral	Inj.	Time	Name	Qty.
☐	☐	....	....	....
☐	☐	....	....	....
☐	☐	....	....	....
☐	☐	....	....	....
☐	☐	....	....	....

❊ Date .... cycle day ⬭ vitamin ⬭ test results ....

Doctor's Instructions:

....

....

....

....

....

....

....

Medications:

Oral	Inj.	Time	Name	Qty.
☐	☐	....	....	....
☐	☐	....	....	....
☐	☐	....	....	....
☐	☐	....	....	....
☐	☐	....	....	....

❊ Date .... cycle day ⬭ vitamin ⬭ test results ....

Doctor's Instructions:

....

....

....

....

....

....

....

Medications:

Oral	Inj.	Time	Name	Qty.
☐	☐	....	....	....
☐	☐	....	....	....
☐	☐	....	....	....
☐	☐	....	....	....
☐	☐	....	....	....

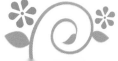

Cycle 1
Week 6

My Thoughts

....
....
....

❈ Date .... cycle day [ ] vitamin [ ] test results ....

Doctor's Instructions:

....
....
....
....
....
....

Medications:

Oral	Inj.	Time	Name	Qty.
☐	☐	....	....	....
☐	☐	....	....	....
☐	☐	....	....	....
☐	☐	....	....	....
☐	☐	....	....	....

❈ Date .... cycle day [ ] vitamin [ ] test results ....

Doctor's Instructions:

....
....
....
....
....
....

Medications:

Oral	Inj.	Time	Name	Qty.
☐	☐	....	....	....
☐	☐	....	....	....
☐	☐	....	....	....
☐	☐	....	....	....
☐	☐	....	....	....

❈ Date .... cycle day [ ] vitamin [ ] test results ....

Doctor's Instructions:

....
....
....
....
....
....

Medications:

Oral	Inj.	Time	Name	Qty.
☐	☐	....	....	....
☐	☐	....	....	....
☐	☐	....	....	....
☐	☐	....	....	....
☐	☐	....	....	....

❋ Date ....

cycle day ☐   vitamin ☐   test results ....

Doctor's Instructions:

....
....
....
....
....
....

Medications:

Oral	Inj.	Time	Name	Qty.
☐	☐	......	....	......
☐	☐	......	....	......
☐	☐	......	....	......
☐	☐	......	....	......
☐	☐	......	....	......

❋ Date ....

cycle day ☐   vitamin ☐   test results ....

Doctor's Instructions:

....
....
....
....
....
....

Medications:

Oral	Inj.	Time	Name	Qty.
☐	☐	......	....	......
☐	☐	......	....	......
☐	☐	......	....	......
☐	☐	......	....	......
☐	☐	......	....	......

❋ Date ....

cycle day ☐   vitamin ☐   test results ....

Doctor's Instructions:

....
....
....
....
....
....

Medications:

Oral	Inj.	Time	Name	Qty.
☐	☐	......	....	......
☐	☐	......	....	......
☐	☐	......	....	......
☐	☐	......	....	......
☐	☐	......	....	......

❋ Date ....

cycle day ☐   vitamin ☐   test results ....

Doctor's Instructions:

....
....
....
....
....
....

Medications:

Oral	Inj.	Time	Name	Qty.
☐	☐	......	....	......
☐	☐	......	....	......
☐	☐	......	....	......
☐	☐	......	....	......
☐	☐	......	....	......

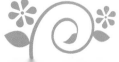

Cycle 1
Reflections

Space
to Vent

Staying Positive

....
....
....
....
....
....
....
....
....
....

It's Worth the Wait

....
....
....
....
....
....
....
....
....
....
....

Cycle 2
Week 1

My Thoughts

....

....

....

❋ **Date** .... cycle day ☐ vitamin ☐ test results ....

Doctor's Instructions:

....

....

....

....

....

....

Medications:

Oral	Inj.	Time	Name	Qty.
☐	☐	....	....	....
☐	☐	....	....	....
☐	☐	....	....	....
☐	☐	....	....	....
☐	☐	....	....	....

❋ **Date** .... cycle day ☐ vitamin ☐ test results ....

Doctor's Instructions:

....

....

....

....

....

....

Medications:

Oral	Inj.	Time	Name	Qty.
☐	☐	....	....	....
☐	☐	....	....	....
☐	☐	....	....	....
☐	☐	....	....	....
☐	☐	....	....	....

❋ **Date** .... cycle day ☐ vitamin ☐ test results ....

Doctor's Instructions:

....

....

....

....

....

....

Medications:

Oral	Inj.	Time	Name	Qty.
☐	☐	....	....	....
☐	☐	....	....	....
☐	☐	....	....	....
☐	☐	....	....	....
☐	☐	....	....	....

❋ Date .... cycle day ⬤ vitamin ⬤ test results ....

Doctor's Instructions:

....
....
....
....
....
....

Medications:

Oral	Inj.	Time	Name	Qty.
☐	☐	......	....	......
☐	☐	......	....	......
☐	☐	......	....	......
☐	☐	......	....	......
☐	☐	......	....	......

❋ Date .... cycle day ⬤ vitamin ⬤ test results ....

Doctor's Instructions:

....
....
....
....
....
....

Medications:

Oral	Inj.	Time	Name	Qty.
☐	☐	......	....	......
☐	☐	......	....	......
☐	☐	......	....	......
☐	☐	......	....	......
☐	☐	......	....	......

❋ Date .... cycle day ⬤ vitamin ⬤ test results ....

Doctor's Instructions:

....
....
....
....
....
....

Medications:

Oral	Inj.	Time	Name	Qty.
☐	☐	......	....	......
☐	☐	......	....	......
☐	☐	......	....	......
☐	☐	......	....	......
☐	☐	......	....	......

❋ Date .... cycle day ⬤ vitamin ⬤ test results ....

Doctor's Instructions:

....
....
....
....
....
....

Medications:

Oral	Inj.	Time	Name	Qty.
☐	☐	......	....	......
☐	☐	......	....	......
☐	☐	......	....	......
☐	☐	......	....	......
☐	☐	......	....	......

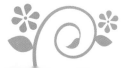

Cycle 2
Week 2

My Thoughts

....

....

....

✿ **Date** .... cycle day ▢ vitamin ▢ test results ....

Doctor's Instructions:

....

....

....

....

....

....

Medications:

Oral	Inj.	Time	Name	Qty.
▢	▢	....	....	....
▢	▢	....	....	....
▢	▢	....	....	....
▢	▢	....	....	....
▢	▢	....	....	....

✿ **Date** .... cycle day ▢ vitamin ▢ test results ....

Doctor's Instructions:

....

....

....

....

....

....

Medications:

Oral	Inj.	Time	Name	Qty.
▢	▢	....	....	....
▢	▢	....	....	....
▢	▢	....	....	....
▢	▢	....	....	....
▢	▢	....	....	....

✿ **Date** .... cycle day ▢ vitamin ▢ test results ....

Doctor's Instructions:

....

....

....

....

....

....

Medications:

Oral	Inj.	Time	Name	Qty.
▢	▢	....	....	....
▢	▢	....	....	....
▢	▢	....	....	....
▢	▢	....	....	....
▢	▢	....	....	....

Date .... cycle day ▢ vitamin ▢ test results ....

Doctor's Instructions:

....
....
....
....
....
....

Medications:

Oral	Inj.	Time	Name	Qty.
▢	▢			
▢	▢			
▢	▢			
▢	▢			
▢	▢			

Date .... cycle day ▢ vitamin ▢ test results ....

Doctor's Instructions:

....
....
....
....
....
....

Medications:

Oral	Inj.	Time	Name	Qty.
▢	▢			
▢	▢			
▢	▢			
▢	▢			
▢	▢			

Date .... cycle day ▢ vitamin ▢ test results ....

Doctor's Instructions:

....
....
....
....
....
....

Medications:

Oral	Inj.	Time	Name	Qty.
▢	▢			
▢	▢			
▢	▢			
▢	▢			
▢	▢			

Date .... cycle day ▢ vitamin ▢ test results ....

Doctor's Instructions:

....
....
....
....
....
....

Medications:

Oral	Inj.	Time	Name	Qty.
▢	▢			
▢	▢			
▢	▢			
▢	▢			
▢	▢			

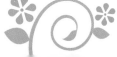

Cycle 2
Week 3

My Thoughts

....
....
....

❋ Date .... cycle day ⬭ vitamin ⬭ test results ....

Doctor's Instructions:

....
....
....
....
....
....

Medications:

Oral	Inj.	Time	Name	Qty.
☐	☐	....	....	....
☐	☐	....	....	....
☐	☐	....	....	....
☐	☐	....	....	....
☐	☐	....	....	....

❋ Date .... cycle day ⬭ vitamin ⬭ test results ....

Doctor's Instructions:

....
....
....
....
....
....

Medications:

Oral	Inj.	Time	Name	Qty.
☐	☐	....	....	....
☐	☐	....	....	....
☐	☐	....	....	....
☐	☐	....	....	....
☐	☐	....	....	....

❋ Date .... cycle day ⬭ vitamin ⬭ test results ....

Doctor's Instructions:

....
....
....
....
....
....

Medications:

Oral	Inj.	Time	Name	Qty.
☐	☐	....	....	....
☐	☐	....	....	....
☐	☐	....	....	....
☐	☐	....	....	....
☐	☐	....	....	....

✿ Date .... cycle day ☐ vitamin ☐ test results ....

Doctor's Instructions:

....
....
....
....
....
....

Medications:

Oral	Inj.	Time	Name	Qty.
☐	☐			
☐	☐			
☐	☐			
☐	☐			
☐	☐			

✿ Date .... cycle day ☐ vitamin ☐ test results ....

Doctor's Instructions:

....
....
....
....
....
....

Medications:

Oral	Inj.	Time	Name	Qty.
☐	☐			
☐	☐			
☐	☐			
☐	☐			
☐	☐			

✿ Date .... cycle day ☐ vitamin ☐ test results ....

Doctor's Instructions:

....
....
....
....
....
....

Medications:

Oral	Inj.	Time	Name	Qty.
☐	☐			
☐	☐			
☐	☐			
☐	☐			
☐	☐			

✿ Date .... cycle day ☐ vitamin ☐ test results ....

Doctor's Instructions:

....
....
....
....
....
....

Medications:

Oral	Inj.	Time	Name	Qty.
☐	☐			
☐	☐			
☐	☐			
☐	☐			
☐	☐			

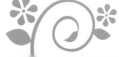

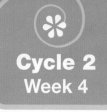

Cycle 2
Week 4

My Thoughts

....
....
....

❋ Date .... cycle day ⬤ vitamin ⬤ test results ....

Doctor's Instructions:

....

....

....

....

....

....

Medications:

Oral	Inj.	Time	Name	Qty.
☐	☐	....	....	....
☐	☐	....	....	....
☐	☐	....	....	....
☐	☐	....	....	....
☐	☐			

❋ Date .... cycle day ⬤ vitamin ⬤ test results ....

Doctor's Instructions:

....

....

....

....

....

....

Medications:

Oral	Inj.	Time	Name	Qty.
☐	☐	....	....	....
☐	☐	....	....	....
☐	☐	....	....	....
☐	☐	....	....	....
☐	☐			

❋ Date .... cycle day ⬤ vitamin ⬤ test results ....

Doctor's Instructions:

....

....

....

....

....

....

Medications:

Oral	Inj.	Time	Name	Qty.
☐	☐	....	....	....
☐	☐	....	....	....
☐	☐	....	....	....
☐	☐	....	....	....
☐	☐			

Date .... cycle day ▢ vitamin ▢ test results ....

Doctor's Instructions:

....

....

....

....

....

....

Medications:

Oral	Inj.	Time	Name	Qty.
▢	▢	.....	.....	.....
▢	▢	.....	.....	.....
▢	▢	.....	.....	.....
▢	▢	.....	.....	.....
▢	▢	.....	.....	.....

Date .... cycle day ▢ vitamin ▢ test results ....

Doctor's Instructions:

....

....

....

....

....

....

Medications:

Oral	Inj.	Time	Name	Qty.
▢	▢	.....	.....	.....
▢	▢	.....	.....	.....
▢	▢	.....	.....	.....
▢	▢	.....	.....	.....
▢	▢	.....	.....	.....

Date .... cycle day ▢ vitamin ▢ test results ....

Doctor's Instructions:

....

....

....

....

....

....

Medications:

Oral	Inj.	Time	Name	Qty.
▢	▢	.....	.....	.....
▢	▢	.....	.....	.....
▢	▢	.....	.....	.....
▢	▢	.....	.....	.....
▢	▢	.....	.....	.....

Date .... cycle day ▢ vitamin ▢ test results ....

Doctor's Instructions:

....

....

....

....

....

....

Medications:

Oral	Inj.	Time	Name	Qty.
▢	▢	.....	.....	.....
▢	▢	.....	.....	.....
▢	▢	.....	.....	.....
▢	▢	.....	.....	.....
▢	▢	.....	.....	.....

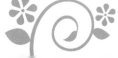

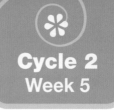

Cycle 2
Week 5

My Thoughts

....
....
....

❋ **Date** .... cycle day ▢ vitamin ▢ test results ....

Doctor's Instructions:

....

....

....

....

....

....

Medications:

Oral	Inj.	Time	Name	Qty.
▢	▢	....	....	....
▢	▢	....	....	....
▢	▢	....	....	....
▢	▢	....	....	....
▢	▢	....	....	....

❋ **Date** .... cycle day ▢ vitamin ▢ test results ....

Doctor's Instructions:

....

....

....

....

....

....

Medications:

Oral	Inj.	Time	Name	Qty.
▢	▢	....	....	....
▢	▢	....	....	....
▢	▢	....	....	....
▢	▢	....	....	....
▢	▢	....	....	....

❋ **Date** .... cycle day ▢ vitamin ▢ test results ....

Doctor's Instructions:

....

....

....

....

....

....

Medications:

Oral	Inj.	Time	Name	Qty.
▢	▢	....	....	....
▢	▢	....	....	....
▢	▢	....	....	....
▢	▢	....	....	....
▢	▢	....	....	....

✤ Date .... cycle day [ ] vitamin [ ] test results ....

Doctor's Instructions:

....

....

....

....

....

....

Medications:

Oral	Inj.	Time	Name	Qty.
☐	☐	....	....	......
☐	☐	....	....	......
☐	☐	....	....	......
☐	☐	....	....	......
☐	☐	....	....	......

✤ Date .... cycle day [ ] vitamin [ ] test results ....

Doctor's Instructions:

....

....

....

....

....

....

Medications:

Oral	Inj.	Time	Name	Qty.
☐	☐	....	....	......
☐	☐	....	....	......
☐	☐	....	....	......
☐	☐	....	....	......
☐	☐	....	....	......

✤ Date .... cycle day [ ] vitamin [ ] test results ....

Doctor's Instructions:

....

....

....

....

....

....

Medications:

Oral	Inj.	Time	Name	Qty.
☐	☐	....	....	......
☐	☐	....	....	......
☐	☐	....	....	......
☐	☐	....	....	......
☐	☐	....	....	......

✤ Date .... cycle day [ ] vitamin [ ] test results ....

Doctor's Instructions:

....

....

....

....

....

....

Medications:

Oral	Inj.	Time	Name	Qty.
☐	☐	....	....	......
☐	☐	....	....	......
☐	☐	....	....	......
☐	☐	....	....	......
☐	☐	....	....	......

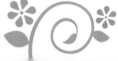

Cycle 2
Week 6

My Thoughts

....

....

....

Date .... cycle day ⬤   vitamin ⬤   test results ....

Doctor's Instructions:

....

....

....

....

....

....

Medications:

Oral	Inj.	Time	Name	Qty.
☐	☐	....	....	....
☐	☐	....	....	....
☐	☐	....	....	....
☐	☐	....	....	....
☐	☐	....	....	....

Date .... cycle day ⬤   vitamin ⬤   test results ....

Doctor's Instructions:

....

....

....

....

....

....

Medications:

Oral	Inj.	Time	Name	Qty.
☐	☐	....	....	....
☐	☐	....	....	....
☐	☐	....	....	....
☐	☐	....	....	....
☐	☐	....	....	....

Date .... cycle day ⬤   vitamin ⬤   test results ....

Doctor's Instructions:

....

....

....

....

....

....

Medications:

Oral	Inj.	Time	Name	Qty.
☐	☐	....	....	....
☐	☐	....	....	....
☐	☐	....	....	....
☐	☐	....	....	....
☐	☐	....	....	....

✻ Date .... cycle day ⬭ vitamin ⬭ test results ....

Doctor's Instructions:

....
....
....
....
....
....

Medications:

Oral	Inj.	Time	Name	Qty.
☐	☐	....	....	....
☐	☐	....	....	....
☐	☐	....	....	....
☐	☐	....	....	....
☐	☐	....	....	....

✻ Date .... cycle day ⬭ vitamin ⬭ test results ....

Doctor's Instructions:

....
....
....
....
....
....

Medications:

Oral	Inj.	Time	Name	Qty.
☐	☐	....	....	....
☐	☐	....	....	....
☐	☐	....	....	....
☐	☐	....	....	....
☐	☐	....	....	....

✻ Date .... cycle day ⬭ vitamin ⬭ test results ....

Doctor's Instructions:

....
....
....
....
....
....

Medications:

Oral	Inj.	Time	Name	Qty.
☐	☐	....	....	....
☐	☐	....	....	....
☐	☐	....	....	....
☐	☐	....	....	....
☐	☐	....	....	....

✻ Date .... cycle day ⬭ vitamin ⬭ test results ....

Doctor's Instructions:

....
....
....
....
....
....

Medications:

Oral	Inj.	Time	Name	Qty.
☐	☐	....	....	....
☐	☐	....	....	....
☐	☐	....	....	....
☐	☐	....	....	....
☐	☐	....	....	....

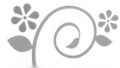

Space
to Vent

Staying Positive

....
....
....
....
....
....
....
....
....
....
....

It's Worth the Wait

....
....
....
....
....
....
....
....
....
....
....

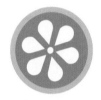

What Now?

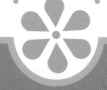

When you began your fertility journey, you didn't want to consider the possibility of months of TTC and more than one cycle of IVF, only to fail to conceive. But, it is a scary reality for some. When IVF and other fertility treatments come up short after several cycles, many couples are completely exhausted — emotionally, physically, and financially. Remember that you don't have to put on a brave front, and especially not for each other. Have a good cry. Failed IVF is a loss worthy of grieving. In time, you will know what the best course of action is.

> "We gain strength, and courage, and confidence by each experience in which we really stop to look fear in the face ... we must do that which we think we cannot."
>
> ~ Eleanor Roosevelt

Many couples find that taking some time off from IVF and beginning again later is the breather they need to regroup and regain their positive perspective. Other couples start researching alternative therapies, such as acupuncture, to assist in conception. Still others look into the adoption process or the possibility of donor eggs or a surrogate mother.

There are many routes to take when the conventional (and even unconventional) methods don't come through. Just relish in the support you and your partner offer each other, and hang in there. Many couples report that they grow much closer after battling infertility and successfully starting a family.

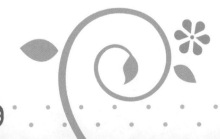

Congratulations!

You're pregnant! The moment you get that confirmation of a positive pregnancy test is undoubtedly one of the happiest moments of your life. All your careful planning and lifestyle changes have paid off!

One of the first questions becomes, who do you tell, and when? Because you can barely contain your excitement, you may want others to share in your joy immediately. Many people will tell only close family members or friends right away. Most couples will wait until the 12-week mark, when the risk for miscarriage drops significantly.

> "My life has been the awaiting you, your footfall was my own heart's beat."
> ~ Paul Valéry

On the other hand, if this pregnancy comes after fertility treatments, you may want to proceed with caution. If you've struggled with infertility or miscarriage in the past, you may want to wait to tell family and friends until you know for certain that the pregnancy is progressing normally.

Next, you will want to continue with the adjustments you made before pregnancy to be sure you and your baby are as happy and healthy as possible. This means continuing with an exercise plan (as approved by your doctor), eating a well-balanced diet, and taking good care of yourself to prevent stress. You will want to learn how to stave off early pregnancy symptoms, like nausea and fatigue. And dad should start figuring out how he can be helpful — for instance, he should take over cleaning the cat's litter box and lifting heavy objects (plus, a foot massage would be nice).

On the following page is an early pregnancy checklist to give you and dad a few important things to think about right away.

Most of all, congratulations on navigating the fertility and conception journey together — and best wishes for your baby on the way!

Early Pregnancy Checklist:

- ☐ Schedule your prenatal doctor's appointment

- ☐ Find a board-certified obstetrician

- ☐ Check with your insurance company to be sure the doctor you have chosen is covered by your plan

- ☐ Call your insurance provider to find out what portion of prenatal visits you will be responsible for

- ☐ Keep taking your prenatal vitamins!

- ☐ Stay hydrated to combat fatigue, but wait to drink water after eating if you are feeling nauseous

- ☐ Cut out foods that give you heartburn or nausea

- ☐ Switch to eating smaller meals more often, instead of three large ones

- ☐ Quit all bad habits cold turkey (if you haven't already), including smoking, drinking alcohol, and taking recreational drugs. No excuses!

- ☐ Check with your doctor to be sure any prescription or over-the-counter medications you are taking are safe

- ☐ Get your doctor's opinion on the safety of caffeine during pregnancy

- ☐ Get a great night's sleep to aid with fatigue

- ☐ Buy pregnancy books and start reading them

- ☐ Work with your doctor to create an exercise plan

- ☐ Start keeping a pregnancy journal or scrapbook

- ☐ Start thinking about baby names

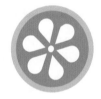

Contacts

Contacts

Use the following pages to record the contact information for anyone helping you on your conception journey.

Name: ....   **Notes:** ....
Title: ....
Company: ....
Address: ....
....
Phone: ....   Cell: ....
Email: ....
Website: ....

Name: ....   **Notes:** ....
Title: ....
Company: ....
Address: ....
....
Phone: ....   Cell: ....
Email: ....
Website: ....

Name: ....   **Notes:** ....
Title: ....
Company: ....
Address: ....
....
Phone: ....   Cell: ....
Email: ....
Website: ....

Name:

Title:

Company:

Address:

Phone: Cell:

Email:

Website:

Notes:

Name:

Title:

Company:

Address:

Phone: Cell:

Email:

Website:

Notes:

Name:

Title:

Company:

Address:

Phone: Cell:

Email:

Website:

Notes:

Name:

Title:

Company:

Address:

Phone: Cell:

Email:

Website:

Notes:

Name: ....

Title: ....

Company: ....

Address: ....

....

Phone: .... **Cell:** ....

Email: ....

Website: ....

Notes: ....

....

....

....

....

....

....

....

Name: ....

Title: ....

Company: ....

Address: ....

....

Phone: .... **Cell:** ....

Email: ....

Website: ....

Notes: ....

....

....

....

....

....

....

....

Name: ....

Title: ....

Company: ....

Address: ....

....

Phone: .... **Cell:** ....

Email: ....

Website: ....

Notes: ....

....

....

....

....

....

....

....

Name: ....

Title: ....

Company: ....

Address: ....

....

Phone: .... **Cell:** ....

Email: ....

Website: ....

Notes: ....

....

....

....

....

....

....

....

Name:	Notes:
Title:	
Company:	
Address:	
Phone: Cell:	
Email:	
Website:	

Name:	Notes:
Title:	
Company:	
Address:	
Phone: Cell:	
Email:	
Website:	

Name:	Notes:
Title:	
Company:	
Address:	
Phone: Cell:	
Email:	
Website:	

Name:	Notes:
Title:	
Company:	
Address:	
Phone: Cell:	
Email:	
Website:	

Name:

Title:

Company:

Address:

Phone: Cell:

Email:

Website:

Notes:

Name:

Title:

Company:

Address:

Phone: Cell:

Email:

Website:

Notes:

Name:

Title:

Company:

Address:

Phone: Cell:

Email:

Website:

Notes:

Name:

Title:

Company:

Address:

Phone: Cell:

Email:

Website:

Notes:

Other Pregnancy & Baby Books
✿ By Alex & Elizabeth Lluch ✿

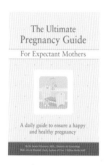

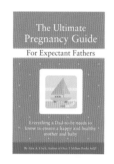

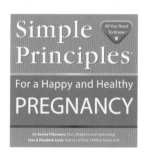

**The Ultimate Pregnancy Guide
For Expectant Mothers**
This comprehensive guide helps
moms-to-be understand what to
expect during pregnancy

US $19.95/Cl., Wire-o
Parenting/Baby
ISBN-13: 978-1-934386-23-1
Size: 7 x 10¼ 262 pp

**The Ultimate Pregnancy Guide
For Expectant Fathers**
This comprehensive guide helps
dads-to-be understand what to
expect during pregnancy

US $19.95/Cl., Wire-o
Parenting/Baby
ISBN-13: 978-1-934386-48-4
Size: 7 x 10¼ 254 pp

**Simple Principles™ for a
Happy and Healthy Pregnancy**
offers 200 pieces of advice that
will help expecting moms have
a safe and stress-free pregnancy

US $9.95/Pb.
Diet & Health/Pregnancy
ISBN-13: 978-1-934386-26-2
Size: 5½ x 5½, 290 pp

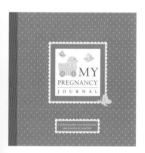

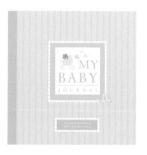

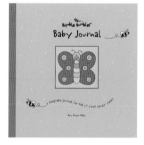

My Pregnancy Journal
This beautiful book is designed
to help expecting mothers
celebrate and reflect on the
exciting journey of pregnancy

US $21.95/Cl., Wire-o
Parenting/Baby
ISBN-13: 978-1-934386-24-8
Size: 10 x 9¼, 100 pp

My Baby Journal
No other baby journal offers so
much to help you preserve the
joy, celebration and development of your baby

US $21.95/Cl., Wire-o
Parenting/Baby
ISBN-13: 978-1-934386-47-7
Size: 9 x 8¾, 100 pp

Humble Bumbles Baby Journal
A National Best-seller!
100 wonderfully illustrated
journal pages that include place-
holders for mementos & more
Designed by: Amy Meyer Allen
US $19.95/Cl., Wire-o
Parenting/Baby
ISBN-13: 978-1-887169-31-8
Size: 9 x 8¾, 100 pp

Visit www.WSPublishingGroup.com to view our extensive line of best-selling books.

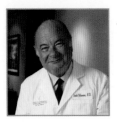

Benito Villanueva, M.D. is an experienced gynecologist and reproductive endocrinologist with more than thirty years exposure to the field of hormone supplementation and replacement. He is an accomplished surgeon with many decades experience of advanced and complex gynecologic surgery, including minimally invasive laparoscopic approach and microsurgery techniques used for fertility restoration.

He has had an illustrious academic career prior to his successful private practice. His obstetrics and gynecology training was at the Georgetown University Medical Center in Washington, D.C., and his reproductive endocrinology and infertility subspecialty training fellowship at the University of Washington in Seattle. He was in the full-time faculty of the University of California-San Diego Medical School in La Jolla for five years prior to creating a very successful medical group, offering state-of-the-art health care in infertility, obstetrics and gynecology.

- Board Certifications: Diplomat, American College of Obstetrics & Gynecology
- Academic Appointments: Department of Reproductive Medicine, UC San Diego School of Medicine, La Jolla, CA
- Reproductive Endocrinology: Clinical Research Fellow, Department of OB/GYN, Division of Reproductive Endocrinology, University of Washington School of Medicine, Seattle, WA
- Residency Training: Department of Obstetrics and Gynecology, Georgetown University Medical Center, Washington, D.C.
- Medical School: National University, Buenos Aires, Argentina

Dr. Villanueva has over 30 years of experience in infertility, obstetrics and gynecology. He resides in La Jolla, California.

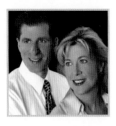

Alex & Elizabeth Lluch are authors of over 3 million books sold in a wide range of categories: health, fitness, diet, home, finance, weddings, children, and babies. Their books are famous for explaining difficult subjects in a clear and easy-to-read manner.

Alex & Elizabeth Lluch have been happily married for over 15 years. They reside in San Diego, California with their three wonderful children.